WHAT CAUSES CANCER?

WHAT WE KNOW AND WHAT IT MEANS

by Anthony B. Miller
MD, FRCP, FRCP(C)

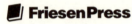 **FriesenPress**

Suite 300 – 852 Fort Street
Victoria, BC, Canada V8W 1H8
www.friesenpress.com

Copyright © 2014 by Anthony B. Miller
First Edition — 2014

This book is dedicated to my wife, Sheena Jessie Miller, without whose support and guidance, it would not have been possible.

Especial thanks also to Dr Paul Kleihues, former Director of the International Agency for Research on Cancer, who conceived the idea for the book, encouraged me to start writing it, and provided me with the means to do so, while I served as Senior Epidemiologist, International Agency for Research on Cancer, January 1998-August 1999.

ISBN
978-1-4602-4675-7 (Hardcover)
978-1-4602-4676-4 (Paperback)
978-1-4602-4677-1 (eBook)

1. Medical, Oncology

Distributed to the trade by The Ingram Book Company

Table of Contents

This book is directed to a broad general audience, in particular those who have already been diagnosed with cancer, as well as their relatives and friends. It is also for those who do not realise that they themselves are at risk for cancer but in practise may be. The central argument of this book is that we know a great deal more about the prevention of cancer than most people realise, and the general public can take many of the actions needed to prevent cancer themselves if they understand what they can do.

The author's career has largely been devoted to research on cancer causes—knowledge that facilitates cancer prevention. His research has also covered cancer screening, but this is often over-valued and prevention is usually by far the better option. He began writing the book while a Senior Scientist at the International Agency for Research on Cancer in Lyon in 2000 and he has revised and extended it over the years.

Introduction

This book is directed to a broad general audience, in particular those who have already been diagnosed with cancer, as well as their relatives and friends. It is also for those who do not realise that they themselves are at risk for cancer but in practise may be.

If you are one of those who have cancer, you are part of a special, but often-neglected group. It is important for you to understand why your cancer occurred; it is increasingly accepted that the factors that cause cancer are often the same ones that encourage cancer to spread. Understanding the cause of your cancer may therefore help you to identify actions that you can take now that could help prevent recurrence and prolong your life. Remember that over two decades ago we were already saying that over half the people that develop cancer would be cured through the right combinations of surgery, radiotherapy, chemotherapy, and hormone therapy. In most developed countries that have good cancer treatment services this proportion is now higher, not only because of improved treatments but also because of increased understanding of the causes of cancer and the resulting lower risk of recurrence these bring. You will also want to know what caused your cancer because of the implications this could have on the risk of cancer among your loved ones, especially your partner, your siblings, and perhaps most significantly, your children.

This book is also especially important for the relatives of people who have cancer. Based on present knowledge there is clear evidence that most cancers are not inherited in the sense that greater risk is passed from parent to child. If you are related to someone with cancer where inherited factors are important you need to know the extent of your own risk and what actions you can take to reduce your risk. However, even for those related to someone with cancer where the risk is not inherited, there are often common factors in the family environment that could increase the risk of cancer in husband or wife, long-term partner, brother and sister, and children. Knowledge of these factors will enable the family to adopt a reduced cancer risk lifestyle for the benefit of all. And indeed, other common chronic diseases share many "risk factors" for cancer, so a lifestyle that reduces the risk of cancer will also reduce the risk of heart disease, respiratory disease and diabetes.

The knowledge of the causes of cancer and, if appropriate action is taken, the reduced risk to families benefits all, not just those who have a family member with cancer. In most countries of the Western world cancer affects about one in three persons in their lifetime. It is not possible yet to tell which person is the one in three, but all three will benefit if they act upon the knowledge that can be obtained from this book and adopt a lifestyle conducive to a reduced cancer risk, in part because of the benefit of reducing the risk of other chronic diseases. Even in developing countries, with growing affluence and longevity, cancer is increasing; there are now few countries in the world where the risk is fewer than one in five adults, and the difference between North and South is rapidly decreasing and may largely disappear by the middle of this century. The causes of this malignant spread from North to South, from the wealthy countries to the poor, are already largely understood. Unfortunately, the knowledge that would enable us to prevent this spread is often not acted upon, either because of lack of understanding, or a refusal by those who do know to act appropriately on the basis of their knowledge. Those of us in the Western world have some responsibility for this lack of action, because it is often our governments or industries that wittingly, for short-term political or economic gains, make policy decisions that have an impact on the cancer risks of other countries, or other generations.

It is hoped that the knowledge you can glean from this book will give you the facts to help to make a difference, and ensure that our governments really do take action that will benefit all humankind. Everyone can and must do something to avoid cancer, by influencing others by example, by helping to disseminate knowledge, and by urging governments to play their part.

The nature of cancer

The term cancer has its origin in a Latin word meaning crab. This exemplifies the characteristics of very advanced, inoperable cancer—as it spreads through the body swollen surface veins can be likened to crab limbs.

The fear of cancer and the idea that having cancer represents a death sentence has been only partly dispelled, even in advanced Western countries, and is still very much part of public understanding on cancer in most developing countries. But as we learn more about how to prevent, detect, and treat cancer effectively, much of this fear is recognised to be misplaced.

The central characteristic that justifies grouping a number of conditions with different causes into one collective called cancer is the multiplication of cells—the microscopic components of our bodies. The basic structure of the cell is that it has a central part, the nucleus, which contains the genetic material that controls the function of the cells, and a surrounding part, the cytoplasm, through which the cell obtains its nutrition, receives oxygen, and discharges carbon dioxide. The nucleus of the cell is critical to cancer development. In humans it contains 23 pairs of chromosomes; these chromosomes contain the genetic material that controls life—deoxyribonucleic acid, or DNA. We term the growths that arise from multiplication of cells "tumours." Tumours can be either benign or malignant. Cancer is a disorder of cell division, and the central characteristic that separates malignant tumours or cancers from benign tumours is the ability to spread, not just locally where the cancer arises (this is also a feature of benign tumours), but also to other parts of the body through the blood and/or lymph systems (metastasise). It is this process of metastasising that makes so many cancers difficult to treat, as local treatment (surgery, or radiotherapy being the prime examples) will not cure the patient. Indeed, it is often the metastases and not the local cancer that kills the patient.

Because cell division is such an integral part of cancer, cancers only occur in tissue that is capable of cell division, a process retained in evolution to preserve the integrity of the body after damage. Cell division is regulated through several checks or balances.Cancers are often described as having completely escaped biological control mechanisms. This is generally true for the highly malignant forms of cancer, but probably not true for the majority of cancers. This is seen in relation to the two most common forms of cancer in women and men—breast and prostate cancer. These two organs are very much under the influence of body control mechanisms, especially the hormones estrogen in women and testosterone in men. This hormonal control is not necessarily lost when cancer occurs in these organs; indeed, several effective forms of cancer treatment are dependent on hormone responsiveness of many of these cancers. A fundamental objective in much cancer research is trying to find what regulates normal cell growth and how that knowledge can be applied to managing cancer. Many scientists dream that they will discover a simple mechanism that will cause normal cell division to be resumed in cancer and thus for the malignant process to cease.

There are two fundamental misconceptions about cancer: that cancer is a disease of civilisation, and that cancers are the result of aging. There is good historical evidence that cancer occurred in antiquity. Some Egyptian mummies and some other human artifacts, especially bones, have been recognised to have signs of cancer. Cancer occurs in animals—indeed, some form of cancer probably occurs in all multicellular beings. Cancer occurs in children, but children are rarely born with cancer. And while it is true that as people age their risk of developing cancer increases, this is not because of aging per se; it is because over time the possibility that someone will encounter a cancer-causing agent increases. Cancer is, therefore, not inevitable. There is also no evidence that cancers are unavoidable. As knowledge increases it has become apparent that the majority of cancers can be prevented, providing the will exists to take the necessary action sufficiently early in life.

Time is very important with regard to cancer. As just indicated, the likelihood that we will encounter a cancer-causing agent increases with time. But time is also important because it takes a long time for cancer to develop—in general it takes years. This is because there are stages of cancer development and the rate that cells pass through the stages is slow. These stages of carcinogenesis (cancer production) are discussed in the next chapter.

Cancers can be classified in two ways—one is by the organ or the tissue from which the cancer arises. (Examples are lung, breast, prostate and skin cancer.) The other way is to base the classification on the appearance of the cancer under the microscope. Examples are leukemia, which arises from the stem cells that form the cells in the blood; lymphomas, which appear to arise from the cells that are responsible for immunity but that can occur in many different organs; and malignant melanoma of the skin, a form of skin cancer that arises from the cells that produce the pigment of the skin that protects against the harmful rays from the sun. For some cancers, these classifications overlap. The nature of the classification used will be described in the chapters on specific cancers that follow.

A popular slogan is that "cancer can be beaten." This can be interpreted to mean that there are some cancers that can be prevented, and some that—with early enough detection and effective treatment—can be cured. Together they comprise about three-quarters of cancers. I prefer to expand the term to mean that the human spirit will not let cancer defeat us, even if incurable. As cancer arises due to errors in an essential aspect of life—the ability of cells to divide and repair injury—it seems unlikely that we shall ever see human-kind completely free of cancer. Even so, we can beat its effects, and for many cancers we can prevent them occurring altogether if we have the will to avoid the exposures that increase their risk.

It was learned many years ago that there are major differences across the world regarding the extent to which cancer occurs. These differences can now be largely explained by the varying extents to which populations are exposed to the factors that cause cancer. Some scientists have taken the genetic differences that can be detected in cancer cells to the point of claiming that cancer occurs because of these genetic differences, and some have gone on to imply that in the future genetic testing will tell us who is destined to develop cancer. However, as knowledge of cancer increases, many have come to recognise that genetic differences account for only a minority of cancers and that it is exposure to external agents through lifestyle, occupation, or environmental factors that explains the majority of cancers. That is good news, because it means that the prevention of the majority of cancers is within grasp, providing we apply the knowledge we have. In the chapters that follow that knowledge and how it can be applied will be explained.

The approaches adopted in this book

Science in cancer research

The two principal sciences that are used to investigate the causes of cancer are epidemiology and basic (laboratory) sciences.

Epidemiology is the science that determines the distribution and determinants (causes) of disease in human populations. As it is impossible to experiment on mankind to find out whether specific agents cause cancer, it is largely an observational science. However, most research within the realm of epidemiology includes the evaluation of means to prevent disease in humans and the types of study can then be of an experimental nature, provided they are carried out with the consent of the subjects concerned. Epidemiology uses statistics as a tool, but its methods extend beyond statistics. To determine the distribution of disease it is necessary to identify the cases that occur in a defined population and in a defined period so that the number of cases per unit of population can be determined. These data are further characterized in terms of age, sex, and sometimes race. For cancer there are two basic types of population data: incidence and mortality. The incidence rate of cancer occurrence is usually expressed as the number of new cases per 100,000 population per year. These figures are derived from population-based cancer registries that have been set up in several areas within countries, and sometimes extended to cover a whole country. Cancer mortality is similarly calculated based on the numbers of deaths from cancer that occur in the defined population in a year. Detailed data on cause of death are obtained from the vital statistics office of the country. Both types of data are coded in accordance with internationally agreed terminology to ensure that data from one country can be compared with data from another. From the incidence and mortality data it is possible to derive estimates of the prevalence of cancer, i.e., the number of cases of the disease that are present in the population at any one time.

Cancer mortality has to be distinguished from the reciprocal of cancer survival, cancer fatality. Cancer mortality is a measure of the death rate from cancer in a population, with the denominator of the rate including people who do and do not have cancer. On the other hand, when deaths from cancer are related to the numbers of people in a group with a specific cancer, we talk of fatality due to cancer. In general, this is not the way people usually discuss this concept—they prefer to discuss the number of people who survive from a cancer and in this book I shall use the term cancer survival to express this. Survival data for cancer are often reported from specific hospitals and calculated over a five-year (or longer) period. Where available, I shall use cancer survival data based not on specific hospitals, but related to all that develop cancer in a population. The longer a patient survives from cancer, the more likely he or she is to be cured. Five-year survival rates are often quoted, as in the past they were almost synonymous with cure. Nowadays, with modern treatments that can maintain reasonable health for many years, survival from cancer has improved, and ten-year survival data may be more realistic.

Cancer epidemiology is not restricted to the descriptive data we have just described. Special studies (often called analytic studies) are also conducted. In cohort studies, a group of people is characterized, and then followed over time to determine and compare the rates of occurrence of cancer according to defined exposures. In case control studies, the previous experience of subjects diagnosed with cancer is compared with that of comparable subjects free of cancer. Both these types of studies, being observational, can involve bias—uncontrollable factors that affect the outcome or distort the inferences drawn from the study. Therefore, before causal conclusions are drawn it is necessary to replicate the findings in other circumstances. Consistency in findings is required before causal conclusions can be drawn.

Data from these studies are referred to frequently in the chapters on specific cancers that follow, although rarely do we find it necessary to refer to the specific type of study that was conducted.

Basic (laboratory) science studies are not affected by the same types of ethical restrictions that affect studies on humans, although for studies that involve intact animals, there are international and national codes for their conduct that are rigorously enforced. Thus, laboratory studies are usually directly experimental rather than observational, with the experimenter going to great pains to control the experimental circumstances and avoid bias. Such studies can be based on intact animals and cells derived from humans or animals, and even extend to the basic molecules that make up cells. As more is learned about the structure and function of normal and cancerous cells, findings show that many biological processes have been conserved during evolution and information gained from studies of one species can be transferred to other species. Although this similarity in function is of great assistance to cancer researchers, it should not be taken too far; we cannot assume that something learned from study of a cell or animal can be applied directly to humans without obtaining some confirmation from a study of humans that confirms that the same mechanisms of action apply.

Much of the conclusions that can be drawn regarding the causes of cancer are based on both epidemiology and basic science research. The two approaches are complementary and I draw heavily on the knowledge gained from them in the chapters that follow.

The natural history of cancer

The process of cancer causation is termed carcinogenesis. The process of carcinogenesis requires years to work through in humans before cancer occurs. It is useful to think of this as a timeline from birth to death. Initially, none of the stages of carcinogenesis have occurred, but the individual is susceptible (sometimes more susceptible than normal because of genetic susceptibility). Then the changes of carcinogenesis begin and a cancer begins to develop. It is not at first detectable, even with the most sophisticated of modern tests, although sometimes immunological changes do occur that may be identified through testing. The cancer then enters a phase where if a sensitive screening test is administered the cancer will be detected; this is called the detectable preclinical phase (DPCP). Regression to normal is still possible during the DPCP, but the longer the cancer persists without regression, the greater the likelihood of progression. With progression of the cancer symptoms occur and the cancer then becomes clinically detectable. If treatment is not successful, death will result.

Mechanisms of cancer causation (carcinogenesis)

Cancer results from the accumulation of multiple (at least two) genetic events within a cell. These genetic changes occur in one or more of the multiple genes in the cell's chromosomes, a process that is called mutation. The reason that two genetic events are required is that the genes occur in pairs, and both members of a pair have to be changed. However, in some familial cancers, one of the relevant genes may have already been transferred from parent to offspring in a changed state so that only one further genetic event may be needed to initiate the process of carcinogenesis, explaining why familial cancers tend to occur earlier in life than spontaneous cancers.

In the past it used to be felt that carcinogenesis occurs in stages, possibly five or more, with three groups of stages generally accepted: initiation, promotion, and progression. Initiation was recognised as a genetic change, occurring when a chemical or physical agent termed a carcinogen came in contact with cells that are sensitive to change. The cells are changed forever, although there may not be any immediate apparent effect on their function or behaviour. If these altered cells come in contact with the second class of agent, a promoter, they begin to change further, and multiply, and cancers may then develop. The third class of agents induce the promoted cells to progress to fully developed invasive cancers, spreading locally and to other organs through the bloodstream or lymph system.

Each of these stages is now recognised as involving changes in the genetic makeup of cells. The temporal sequence of the genetic events varies among tissues and cells. The selection of cells with genetic mutations crucial to cancer development results in cell multiplication to produce a population of identical cells, or a clone that eventually gives rise to a tumour. Successive genetic changes may give rise to a series of clones, each one with an advantage over its predecessors so that eventually the tumour occurs. There may be several years between each of these steps, as the probability that the individual will encounter the agent or carcinogen that induces the next step will increase with time. Each successive clone is more likely to represent the final cancer. Cellular division, which increases the probability that mistakes will occur and that new clones will develop, is clearly essential. But this may not be the only mechanism. The body is able to recognise cells that change, and if they appear to be very unusual (and potentially dangerous), cell death, or apoptosis, may be induced. Further selection against apoptosis may be one of the main mechanisms that leads to the development of cancer.

This process takes many years, and these changes are very much conditioned by stochastic or chance events. There is considerable evidence that the target genes of genetic changes relevant to cancer are "cell-cycle prone," that is, their sensitivity to change depends on whether the cell is in a resting or active growth phase. The growth and spread of cancer is also determined by alterations of the organisational society of cell populations. The alteration of expression of the relevant cancer-causing genes (oncogenes), or relaxation of the function of tumour suppressor genes, either through mutations or non-mutational processes, is largely determined by environmental factors.

The proper designation of a carcinogen requires experimental (basic) studies, usually on laboratory animals. Rodents (especially mice and rats) are often used for this purpose, although other animal species, such as hamsters, dogs, and sometimes primates are used as well. However, even if sufficient evidence of carcinogenicity is obtained in animals, this is only an indication of potential effects in humans. This is, in part, because of species differences, and in part because many carcinogens in animals have been identified using levels of exposure far in excess of that likely to be experienced by humans.

To establish that an animal carcinogen is a human carcinogen requires epidemiological studies in humans. Epidemiology can help bring understanding to the process of carcinogenesis in terms of the time relationships of exposure and cancer occurrence. Epidemiologists tend to use the terms "early-stage" and "late-stage" carcinogenesis. Increasingly, epidemiologists are collaborating with basic scientists to incorporate markers of genetic changes in epidemiology studies. This facilitates further understanding of the processes of human carcinogenesis.

The concept of risk

The term "risk" is used frequently in the sections that follow. The average risk of developing cancer over the next year for people living within a certain area is best defined by the incidence rate of the cancer. For example, a white woman age between 50 and 54 living in the US will have a risk of developing breast cancer in the next year of 220 per 100,000, which translates into a risk over the next five years of 11 per 1,000, or just over 1 per 100.

Such data can be cumulated over the lifetime (to age 75, for example) to give an estimate of lifetime risk. For white women in the US, for example, the cumulative risk to age 75 is about 10%, i.e., one in 10 women who survive to that age will develop breast cancer. This is not the same as one in every 10 women born, as that calculation ignores the fact that not all women survive to age 75, but it is useful nevertheless as it gives an indication of the relative importance of various cancers in a form that may be understood by the people who are at risk.

Although cumulative risk is readily understood and interpreted within countries, it is less useful for comparisons between countries. Under these circumstances it is more usual to make comparisons of incidence or mortality across a lifetime that are corrected for the different age structure of the associated populations. These age-corrected or age-standardized rates are themselves an indication of risk and can be readily used to compare risk between different countries, or even areas within countries. The calculations require selection of a standard population, and conventionally, when comparing cancer incidence and mortality, a population resembling that of the world as a whole is used.

It is often easier to understand the relative importance of different cancers by presenting the amount they contribute to the total in terms of percentages.

In every population the degree of risk varies according to the extent people have been exposed to cancer-causing substances. The risk of developing lung cancer in a heavy smoker is about 20 times the risk in a non-smoker, while the risk of developing colon cancer in someone who eats plenty of fruits and vegetables is about half the risk of someone who eats few fruits or vegetables. These are relative risks (e.g., the risks among smokers relative to the risks among non-smokers) and are expressed in units or fractions of a unit. A relative risk (RR) of 1.0 implies no increased risk, a risk of 2.0 a doubling of risk and of 0.5 a halving of risk. Cancer-causing factors therefore give rise to relative risks greater than 1.0, while cancer preventive factors to relative risks less than 1.0.

One other descriptor of risk that I shall also use is the attributable risk—the amount of cancer that is considered to be caused by a specific factor. I shall usually use the term in relation to the population—the percentage of cancer in a population caused by the factor. For example, in all countries that have succumbed to the tobacco epidemic, about 80% of lung cancer is caused by tobacco smoking.

Sometimes several factors work together to cause cancer in the individual and often these attributable risks overlap. Therefore, we should not expect attributable risk factors to add to exactly 100%—the total may be considerably more, especially if we know a great deal about multiple causes of a cancer. However, the extent of our knowledge about causes of specific cancers can be gauged by the extent to which the attributable risks add to 100% or more.

Associations, risk factors and causes

When the presence or absence of a factor, such as a chemical, or variations in the amount of a factor, such as a constituent of diet, is found to correlate with variation in the occurrence of a cancer, an association is said to have been demonstrated. A factor that is associated with cancer occurrence may be a cause of cancer, but it may also be a marker of a true cause with which it is itself associated and which may or may not have been studied—in that case the factor is not a cause, but is regarded as a confounder of the true cause.

Factors that are found to be associated with cancer occurrence or risk are often termed "risk factors" if it is not certain that they are true causes, or if it is known that they are not. An example of the latter is social class, or socio-economic status (SES). SES is often found to be associated with cancer occurrence. But it is not the cause of the cancer; some factor (or factors) that varies with SES is the true cause, such as exposure to carcinogenic chemicals in occupation, differences in tobacco use, and differences in diet and nutrition.

A cause of cancer is defined as a factor that increases the probability that cancer will develop in an individual. Conversely, it can also be operationally defined as a factor, the removal of which decreases the occurrence of a cancer in a population. Given that causes of cancer can be evaluated in experimental animals, tests on animals for carcinogenicity play a major role in assessing whether a factor is a cause of cancer. But to be certain that the factor is important in causing cancer in a human population it is necessary for epidemiology studies to be conducted. These have to demonstrate that chance or confounding can be discounted as explanations for the associations seen. Indeed, only epidemiology can determine if removal of a factor reduces the occurrence of cancer in a population. In the chapters that follow I shall distinguish between known causes and suspected causes. Where factors have been suggested to be causes but where the evidence is non-existent, or the evidence shows it is extremely unlikely to be the factor causes that cancer, I shall sometimes refer to them as "unknown" causes.

The types of causes of cancer

GENES (HEREDITY)

As implied above, cancer is induced by genetic changes in cells, possibly even a single cell, which then divides and multiplies to form a mass of identical cells (a clone). Indeed, several genetic changes have to occur for a cancer to develop. However, that does not mean that all cancers are hereditary, with the genetic predisposition passed from parent to offspring. It is now clear that, although some cancers are hereditary, the proportion of common cancers that are hereditary, such as breast, lung, and colon cancers, is only in the order of 5% to 10%. For some relatively rare cancers, such as retinoblastoma of the eye, the proportion that is hereditary is much larger. Further, there are some rare inherited conditions with a marked predisposition to cancer. These are so uncommon, however, that I shall not be discussing them in this book. However, I shall discuss for every cancer considered the evidence that is currently available on genetic predisposition and inheritance of cancer. Perhaps the most important message at this stage is for the reader to recognize that in general cancer is not a hereditary disease.

INFECTIOUS AGENTS

Cancer is also not an infectious disease, by which we mean that contact with someone who has cancer will not induce cancer in the person free of cancer. However, that does not imply that there are no infectious causes of cancer. Indeed, it is now clear that some viruses are direct causes of certain cancers. There are two common cancers in developing countries that are virus-induced: cancer of the liver and cancer of the uterine cervix, as well as several other less common cancers. The prevention of liver cancer by vaccination against the hepatitis B virus is almost certainly achievable. Vaccination against the human papilloma viruses that cause cancer of the cervix is now possible. Perhaps as much as 15% of all cancers are caused by viruses. But again, I emphasize that although the viruses are passed from human to human to eventually cause a cancer in some of those infected (usually as a result of chronic infection in a minority of those infected), that does not mean that the person with the cancer is infectious.

There is one virus that increases the risk of cancer in those infected, but the mechanism appears to be immunosuppression, rather than carcinogenicity, and that is the Human Immunodeficiency Virus (HIV), the cause of Acquired Immunodeficiency Syndrome (AIDS). The risk of an otherwise rare sarcoma (Kaposi's sarcoma), lymphomas, and cancer of the uterine cervix are increased in those infected with the HIV virus. I shall give more details later in the relevant chapters.

There are some other biological agents that increase the risk of cancer. One is the bacterium *Helicobacter pylori*, a cause of stomach cancer. Another is a human parasite found in North Africa, *Schistosoma haematobium*, which increases the risk of bladder cancer. Again, these are discussed further in the relevant sections that follow.

CHEMICALS, INCLUDING TOBACCO

There are a large number of chemicals known to cause cancer. By far the most important in terms of the damage wrought to human health are the collections of chemicals in tobacco smoke. In developed countries 30% of cancers in men are caused by tobacco, and the percentage in women in developed countries—and, tragically, in both men and women in developing countries—is rising rapidly.

Several chemicals have been recognized to be carcinogenic as a result of relatively high exposure to humans under occupational circumstances and subsequent evaluation of the risk of cancer in comparison to an unexposed group. Others have been identified as probably carcinogenic to humans as a result of experiments in animals. Animal tests of carcinogenicity cannot be used to predict more than a probability that a substance will be carcinogenic to humans. Animal tests are done on relatively small numbers of animals, often in groups of 50-90. In order to detect a carcinogenic effect, chemicals usually have to be tested at very high doses, very close to their maximum tolerated dose, just below the level that will kill the animal from toxicity. They are also usually tested in rodents, and the metabolism of rodents is not identical to man. The routes of administration also vary. Finally, the site that a cancer occurs in excess in a rodent is not necessarily the same as what occurs in man. Dogs are better predictors of site-specific carcinogenesis, and primates are even better. But because of the expense of such tests, tests for carcinogenicity in dogs are performed infrequently, and tests in primates are rarely performed.

As a result of many years experience with evaluating the carcinogenicity of chemicals in humans, the International Agency for Research on Cancer (IARC) of the World Health Organization (WHO) has established criteria to assess the likelihood that a chemical or other agent is carcinogenic to humans. These evaluations are published on a regular basis. I shall draw heavily on these evaluations in this book in relation to the relevant cancer sites in humans, but will tend to concentrate on the chemicals characterised as carcinogenic to humans (group 1). Where exposure is high, or there is substantial interest in the chemical, I shall also refer to chemicals evaluated as probably carcinogenic to humans (group 2A), or possibly carcinogenic to humans (group 2B). Readers interested in the evaluation of the carcinogenicity of a particular chemical should consult the relevant volume in the IARC *Monograph* series. (The monographs can be accessed via the website: monographs.iarc.fr.)

PHYSICAL AGENTS

Some physical agents, such as ionizing radiation (e.g., X-rays and exposure to gamma rays through uranium mining), and non-ionizing radiation (sunlight) are causes of some cancers. I shall consider these in relation to the relevant cancer sites, for example, lung, skin, etc.

DIET

The human diet is extremely complex, and it has departed a long way from the diet at the time of the origin of man in evolutionary terms, when mankind belonged to simple hunter/gatherer societies. Diet appears to include factors that both increase the risk of cancer, and factors that reduce it. Diet is difficult to study epidemiologically. Individuals can usually recall what they ate recently and make a good stab at reporting their usual diet, but are often unable to describe in sufficient detail the diet they had in the past. Indeed, there is a tendency to describe past diet in terms of what people eat now, rather than the true diet of the past. Yet it is the past diet, rather than the present diet that we need to evaluate in regard to cancer causation. There are even more difficulties. Even if the diet of a large number of people is characterized now, and they are followed forward in time to determine their risk of cancer in relation to the diet they eat at the time we commenced studying them, they may change their diet in ways that could influence cancer occurrence, or their diet may have been recorded too late in the process of cancer causation to correctly relate the dietary factors measured to the occurrence of cancer.

As a result of these uncertainties, it is often not possible to state with confidence which specific dietary factors are causes of cancer, although we have many clues that I shall discuss below. Even so, it seems likely that dietary factors are among the most important, and perhaps the most important, factors in cancer occurrence, and that they account for approximately 20% of all cancers in the world.

ALCOHOL

Alcohol is one factor in human diet that is recorded fairly accurately by humans, providing the right (confidential) approach is made to them. High alcohol intake has been found to be associated with increased risk of cancer of a number of cancer sites, some in association with smoking, but some as alcoholic beverages alone. The evidence was sufficiently strong that, as early as 1988, IARC categorized the drinking of alcoholic beverages as carcinogenic to humans. Often it is not clear which of the many alcoholic beverages are carcinogenic, although when studied nearly all seem to increase the risk of one or another cancer to some extent. I shall discuss such evidence in the relevant chapters that follow.

PHYSICAL ACTIVITY

There is increasing evidence that physical activity, even to a moderate degree, reduces the risk of some cancers, especially some of those associated with diet. This possibly represents a better use of energy intake, itself suspected as influencing the risk of some cancers. As for diet, I shall discuss the evidence in relation to specific cancer sites.

Meaning of the environment

The environment of humans is generally considered as everything external to mankind. However, it is useful to consider the environment in two groupings: the general and the personal.

THE GENERAL ENVIRONMENT

The general environment includes the air humans breathe, the water they drink, the land on which they live and work, the climatic conditions they encounter, and the pollution that enters these spaces. Overall, humans are not in direct control of the general environment and personal actions, other than simply moving or migrating elsewhere, can do little to ameliorate whatever carcinogenic or other hazard to health may be present in the general environment. The public usually refer to the general environment when they refer to the causes of disease, such as cancer, and I shall do the same in this book to avoid confusion. There is often controversy as to the amount of cancer caused by the general environment. In part this is because epidemiologists have popularized the well-founded statement that 80% of cancer is caused by environmental factors, a statement that has to be interpreted as including the personal environment, which present evidence shows is far more responsible for cancer occurrence than the general environment as defined here. However, there is also the difficulty of studying the causes of cancer in relation to the general environment, when the factors of interest are distributed widely and found in low concentrations. In practice the methods to study cancer risk in relation to such exposures are not well developed, and controversy flourishes when dogma replaces scientific fact. All that can be stated with certainty at present is that the proportion of cancer as a whole due to contamination of the general environment is probably rather low, some have estimated not more than 1% to 2%.

THE PERSONAL ENVIRONMENT

In contrast to the general environment, individuals have control of their personal environment, which consists of the substances people eat and drink, whether they smoke or allow themselves to be exposed to the smoke of others, whether they sunbathe, and what they bring into their homes. Two of these factors, smoking and diet, are believed to account for well over half of all cancers—nearer 70%

in developed countries—and therefore the large majority of cancers are influenced by, and potentially prevented by, individual human action. It would be confusing to refer to these factors as "environmental," so I shall not use the term "personal environment" further in this book, but instead refer to the individual factors that comprise it.

Cancer prevention

PERSONAL ACTIONS

As just implied, individuals who decide to not smoke and to consume a nutritious, well-balanced diet, without excess intake of animal fat and with adequate consumption of fruits and vegetables, can do much to reduce their risk of cancer, especially if action occurs relatively early in life. Additional personal actions that will reduce the risk of cancer include avoiding excess alcohol intake, undertaking physical exercise on a regular basis, and being aware of the substances used in connection with one's occupation and avoiding contact with those that are hazardous. It is no accident that most of these actions are recommended for reduction in risk of cardiovascular disease. Cardiovascular disease and cancer share many of the same risk factors; actions taken to reduce the risk of these chronic conditions are often identical.

ACTIONS BY GOVERNMENT

Governments can facilitate cancer prevention in a number of ways. Raising the taxes on tobacco products, and ensuring that agricultural practices are supportive of healthy diets will help to facilitate personal cancer preventive actions. Regulations concerning testing of new chemicals for carcinogenicity before their use is permitted and regulating, if not abolishing, exposure of workers to hazardous substances will reduce occupational cancer. Actions by governments to reduce pollution of the general environment may also help to prevent some cancers. Actions by governments are often dictated by short-term economic and/or political considerations.

Governments should be conscious of the need to maintain the health of the populations they serve and also raise the profile of health in decision making.

RELATIONSHIP OF PREVENTION TO
SCREENING AND TREATMENT

Prevention, screening, and treatment are the main planks of cancer control. Prevention, if it can be achieved, is preferable, as the costs associated with occurrence of the disease—economic, physical, and psychological—will simply not be incurred. However, prevention may not be feasible, either because of lack of knowledge of the causes, or because the preventive action necessary would have too many undesirable consequences to adopt as a matter of policy. Further, the long natural history of cancer may make it impossible to introduce preventive actions to prevent all cancers in the current generation, the main impact being too delayed, and therefore such action may largely benefit subsequent generations. For these reasons, where early detection followed by effective therapy has been shown to reduce cancer mortality, such approaches must form an important component of cancer control.

For these reasons, in the sections that follow I shall discuss secondary prevention, or screening, where it has been shown to be effective in relation to specific cancer sites. However, I shall not consider therapy, as this would not be compatible with the objectives of this volume.

Chapter 1

Breast Cancer

It is a striking feature of breast cancer that it is clearly not a modern disease, as many indications of breast cancer in women depicted in the art of former times demonstrate. Breast cancer is derived from the "glandular" cells of the breast—those cells that form the primary structure within the breast that are responsible for lactation. This complicated structure of microscopic sacs and passages that gradually join to form a system of ducts to empty at the nipple develops during puberty, but does not attain its full maturity until the time of first completed pregnancy. The whole length of this system, from the milk sacs to the ducts at the nipple is susceptible to the development of cancer. Many cancers, however, appear to first develop in the smaller ducts. The supportive fibrous and fatty tissues that make up the breast are not the source of breast cancer. Occasionally some benign tumours develop in this supportive structure, sometimes in younger women, and very occasionally in older women malignant tumours of the fibrous tissue develop. The causes of these rare tumours are not known; in the following sections I restrict my attention to the common glandular cancers.

Pathologists call the majority (about 70%) of invasive cancers of the breast "ductal carcinoma," although it is not clear that they all necessarily arise within ducts. Another 20% are called "invasive lobular cancer," and the remaining medullary, mucous producing adenocarcinomas, and rarer types. Although this has not been established, these different types may have some relationship to the causes of breast cancer, except that medullary breast cancers appear to be associated with a positive family history of breast cancer.

Increasingly, gene products are being used to distinguish different types of breast cancer that may respond to a different extent to various treatments. Generally, these types are diagnosed by the presence or absence of three gene receptors: estrogen receptor (ER), progesterone receptor (PR), and human epidermal growth factor receptor 2 (HER2). When tests for each of these receptors are negative (i.e., the receptors are not detectable in the cancer cells), the cancer is called "triple negative."

Triple negative breast cancer accounts for approximately 15% of all invasive breast cancers and most commonly affects younger patients, women of African, Latina or Caribbean descent, and carriers of the BRCA1 gene. (For further information on the BRCA1 gene, please see below.) These cancers require more complicated treatment than other forms of breast cancer, otherwise they have a relatively poor survival.

In developed countries such as Canada, the UK, and the US, the risk of developing breast cancer increases steadily throughout life; as women age they become at greater risk of developing breast cancer than at earlier times in their life. Breast cancer is a rare disease in young women. But even in the highest risk white population of North America (in their eighties), breast cancer occurs in only about 20 women per 1,000 or 2% over the ensuing five-year period. In most countries, breast cancer occurs in over 100 women to every man. In Japan, incidence remains level from about the age of 45. This is similar to the effect seen in many other Asian and developing countries. This is an indication that the risk of breast cancer in Japan will increase, and that as young women age their risk could become more closely aligned to that in North America and Europe.

While breast cancer is the most common cancer in women in the world (in developed and developing regions) it is not the commonest cause of death from cancer in women—that distinction is now held by lung cancer. The causes of breast cancer are not as well understood in men as in women, and most of the following discussion relates to women. Breast cancer is rare in men, but it does occur. Where there is specific information on men, I provide it.

Breast cancer is associated with relative affluence, and therefore is commoner in Western countries than those of the developing world, but in Western countries all women are at risk, although within these countries there are different degrees of risk. In North America currently it is commonly stated that breast cancer occurs in about one in nine women; in other Western countries the risk is about one in 10 to 14. These figures are based on the concept of lifetime risk, discussed in the introduction to this book. This does not mean that one of every nine women born will develop breast cancer; it means that as women age they gradually accumulate this degree of risk, but it does not reach the one in nine level until they survive to their eighties.

For younger women, the risk reaches 20 per 1,000 by age 50 in North America, which translates to a risk of one in 50.

The range of mortality rates is much lower because of the more favourable survival of breast cancer in (high-incidence) developed regions. The highest mortality rates are in Northern Europe and Northern Africa. However, rates in Asia are the lowest in the world for both incidence and mortality. Breast cancer ranks as the fifth cause of death from cancer overall in the world (458,000 deaths), but it is still the most frequent cause of cancer death in women in developing countries (269,000 deaths or 12.7% of total) and nearly all developed regions, where the estimated 189,000 deaths is almost equal to the estimated number of deaths from lung cancer (188,000 deaths). Death rates from lung cancer now exceed those from breast cancer in Canada and the US.

Breast cancer is increasing in incidence in all areas of the world, both in developed countries and in countries that are moving along the path of development. In most developing countries breast cancer is not the commonest cancer in women; that place is taken by cancer of the uterine cervix. But as countries make the economic transition to relative wealth, almost invariably they make the epidemiological transition to a country where breast cancer is more common than cervix cancer.

Increasing awareness of the importance of breast cancer, with the promotion of earlier and better diagnosis, was probably responsible for some of the increases in breast cancer in many Western countries in recent decades. More recently, use of screening mammography and hormone replacement therapy has also contributed to the rising rates of breast cancer that have been experienced in most Western countries. Screening brings forward the time of diagnosis of breast cancer, and may bring to light cancers that might never have been detected in some women. This increases the incidence of breast cancer at the ages screening is now occurring, especially over the age of 50, but in some countries, including the US, from the age of 40. This is what we call over-diagnosis—cancers that had reached their stage of maximum growth, probably because of the action of body defence mechanisms, and would never have become apparent were it not for screening. This needs to be borne in mind in interpreting trends in the incidence of breast cancer; countries that introduced mammography screening showed major increases in the incidence of breast cancer, but this should be interpreted as an artifact of screening, not an indication that the risk of breast cancer is increasing.

Deaths from breast cancer are also increasing in many countries. Those countries with lower rates in the 1950s (for example, Japan and Finland) show consistent increases in mortality, although for Finland the increase ceased around 1990, and a small decline occurred thereafter. Canada and the US showed almost stable mortality until 1990 when a substantial fall began. Denmark and especially the UK showed important increases, but from 1990 a substantial decline has occurred at the same rate for Canada and the US. Sweden showed stability, then a slow decline from about 1970.

Interpretation of these trends is difficult. Most of the increases are reflections of the increase in incidence. Most of the recent decreases are probably due to improvements in the outcome of therapy for breast cancer, a reflection of the gains achieved through adjuvant chemotherapy and hormonal therapy in clinical trials being applied in practice in the general population. Some consider part of the recent falls in Canada, the UK, and the US to be due to the success of screening programs. The programs in Canada began too recently to explain the mortality reduction, while the slow fall in Sweden suggests that the extensive screening there may not have had much impact; adoption of adjuvant treatment in Sweden later than in Canada and the US may explain the lesser reduction. A further discussion of these contrasting explanations for the falls in breast cancer mortality will be found in the section on Secondary Prevention toward the end of this chapter.

The prognosis of breast cancers relates a little to their type, as discussed earlier, but more directly corresponds to their size when detected—the larger the cancer the poorer the outcome. Prognosis also relates to whether the cancer can be shown to have spread to regional lymph nodes, especially in the axilla—the larger the number of nodes involved by the cancer the worse the outcome. Other prognostic factors include the grade of the cancer, particularly dependent on characteristics of their nuclei, and whether the cancer can be shown to have hormone receptors, (estrogen or progesterone); those that are hormone receptor positive have a better outcome.

For the average woman diagnosed with an invasive breast cancer in North America the chance of survival to five years is at least 80%, and to ten years 60% or more. The five-year relative survival for breast cancer (relative to the survival of those free from breast cancer of similar age) during 2002-2008 from 18 US areas was 89%. In Canada five-year relative survival increased from 82% in

1992-1994 to 88% in 2005-2007. For women diagnosed with in situ breast cancer, an almost 100% survival is the rule. However, if a woman has a very advanced breast cancer that has already spread to other organs the chance of survival for five years is less than 30%. This tends to be reflected in poorer survival in some developing countries as compared to many developed nations. One study has suggested that the relative survival of breast cancers diagnosed in the late 1980s in developing countries ranged from 45% to 70%, but was only 12.5% in the Gambia in Africa.

The early stages of breast cancer, before the cancer begins to spread within the breast, are largely undetectable, even on mammography. However, it is believed that in the lining of the smaller ducts the cells can change in response to cancer-causing stimuli, and eventually these changes are recognizable through their proliferation, within the ducts and sometimes the milk sacs. These proliferative masses are called atypical hyperplasia and they are sometimes detected serendipitously in a woman who has a piece of the breast removed because of a suspicion of breast cancer.

Another stage that some believe is a precursor of invasive breast cancer is called carcinoma in situ. This is non-invasive cancer, the commonest varieties being called intraductal because they seem to develop within ducts. Intraductal carcinomas in situ may come to light accidentally, but more often are recognized because the inner part of these collections of cells tends to die, or necrose, and within this necrosis characteristic fine calcifications develop that are detectable on mammography. Some of these intraductal tumours may become extensive within the breast, and they may sometimes be associated with the early signs of invasion. It is these types that may eventually become invasive cancers. However, it is unlikely that carcinomas in situ invariably become invasive, or malignant; rather, the majority appear to be markers of future risk of invasive cancer. The majority of invasive cancers of the breast occur in women who have not been found previously to have either atypical hyperplasia or carcinoma in situ.

Breast cancers usually take a long time to develop. It has been estimated that the "doubling time" of breast cancers—the time it takes for cancers to double in size—is on average about 90 days. This is relatively slow growth compared to many other cancers. This means that the time before a cancer becomes detectable, if the right tests are applied, can be several years, and for many cancers, the time from initial commencement to diagnosis with symptoms as long as 10 or more years. Breast cancer, therefore, compared to many other cancers, has a long natural history, and although the risk of recurrence after initial successful treatment of breast cancer declines over the next five years, breast cancers can still recur as long as 20 years after diagnosis.

Proven causes of breast cancer

CHEMICAL AGENTS
EXOGENOUS HORMONES

Breast cancer is called a hormonally dependent cancer—that is, it comes under the influence of natural (or endogenous) estrogens. Therefore, it would not be surprising if risk of breast cancer was affected by the use of oral contraceptives and non-contraceptive estrogens, usually taken for relief of menopausal symptoms and often called estrogen replacement therapy. For a while this was controversial, but after numerous studies, a consensus emerged.

It now seems clear that women who took oral contraceptives for at least five years 20 or more years ago to delay first pregnancy or space pregnancies have about a 50% increase in risk of breast cancer (relative risk 1.5). Because of the age of these women, the increase in risk appears to have begun in their 30s and to continue at least through their 40s. An additional group of women who took oral contraceptives when they were in their 40s appear to have been at increased risk of breast cancer while they took oral contraceptives.

Most of the preparations of oral contraceptives used 20 years ago had a higher dose of estrogens than has been common recently. It is uncertain whether the newer low-dose estrogen preparations will have the same effect in increasing breast cancer risk as the older preparations. It is also uncertain whether women who took the older high-estrogen dose preparations will show the same increase in breast cancer risk as they enter their 50s and 60s.

Studies of the effect of the injectable contraceptive, medroxy-progesterone acetate (Provera), indicate that this preparation, free of estrogen, also increases breast cancer risk by a similar extent as for oral contraceptives, with an effect that begins immediately after the first injection. The mechanism of this effect is uncertain, but it confirms that the effects of various hormones on breast cancer are not entirely due to estrogen-like actions.

Non-contraceptive estrogens are now accepted as increasing the risk of breast cancer. This effect is detectable after about a five-year period of use and tends to affect largely the risk of breast cancer in women in their 60s. Again, the increase in risk is in the order of 50%. The increase in risk persists while the estrogens are being taken, but appears to cease within about five years after their use has stopped. There is some evidence that the types of breast cancers found in women taking non-contraceptive estrogens have a better outcome than those not taking estrogens.

There are many benefits of hormonal replacement therapy in women over and above the effects in reducing menopausal symptoms, including a beneficial effect in reducing the risk of osteoporosis. Thus, although these agents also increase the risk of endometrial cancer (cancer of the uterus), it is probable that the overall health benefit for women offsets the increase in risk of cancer. However, this is something that the individual woman has to decide, guided by her physician.

ALCOHOL

The possibility that high alcohol consumption increases the risk of breast cancer was raised many years ago. Since then many studies have been conducted to unravel this association. Although some were negative, the vast majority have confirmed increasing breast cancer risk with higher alcohol consumption, with risk increased by about 20% to 50% with as little as one glass of wine a day. The heavier the consumption, the greater the risk. The type of alcohol consumed does not seem to be important, although in most studies the majority of alcohol consumed was wine.

Early on it was assumed that alcohol consumption was acting as a marker of some other aspect of lifestyle, perhaps particularly diet. However, several of the studies collected dietary consumption as well as alcohol consumption data, and the alcohol effect appears to be independent of diet, as it is of other breast cancer risk factors. Why alcohol should increase breast cancer risk is uncertain, although it does not seem to be an estrogen effect, but rather a direct effect of alcohol metabolites in increasing cancer development.

TOBACCO SMOKING

Smoking is now recognized as increasing the risk of breast cancer, especially prolonged smoking that begins in the period before the first pregnancy. The increased risk from active smoking is paralleled by increased risk of passive smoking (environmental tobacco smoke), especially in pre-menopausal women. Tobacco smoking seems to have a greater effect in increasing the risk of breast cancer in those who are genetically susceptible to the disease.

PHYSICAL AGENTS

Ionizing radiation is an established cause of breast cancer, demonstrated particularly in follow-up studies of women who received radiation as a result of the atomic bomb explosions in Hiroshima and Nagasaki, and the follow up of women who were exposed to high levels of radiation to the chest during the pre-chemotherapy era for treatment of tuberculosis. In the latter group radiation was not given directly for the treatment of tuberculosis, rather it was a consequence of multiple fluoroscopic X-ray examinations to control the amount of air inserted into the chest cavity to put the affected lung at rest.

Both of these sets of studies have demonstrated that even the prepubertal breast is susceptible to the effects of ionizing radiation and that susceptibility lasts until about the age of first completed pregnancy and birth. Thereafter risk falls substantially, so that women who receive irradiation to their breasts in the late 30s or 40s have only a fraction of the risk of breast cancer compared to women irradiated earlier in life. This has made it possible to determine that the risk to women from radiation from mammography given after the age of 40 is extremely low.

Radiation given to the pelvis damages the ovaries and will reduce the risk of breast cancer. This is because of the inhibitory effect on estrogen production, as discussed in more detail later. (See reproductive behaviour, below.)

DIET AND NUTRITION

Nearly every study investigating diet and breast cancer has found that excess caloric intake is associated with increased breast cancer risk. What is more controversial is whether the nature of the energy contained in foods is important, and particularly whether a high intake of fat, the most energy-dense nutrient, is the prime culprit. Some of the early animal studies that suggested a role of dietary fat consumption in increasing the risk of mammary cancer were followed by human studies that suggested the same relationship. However, this became confused when it was realized that in Mediterranean countries, where the intake of fats is quite high, although largely of the monounsaturated fat in olive oil, breast cancer risk tended to be lower than in countries where the dominant fat consumed was fat of animal origin, usually saturated fats. More recent studies that have attempted to find an energy-independent role of fat in increasing breast cancer risk have largely been negative, but it is still possible that if the energy content of the diet, and particularly if the intake of saturated fats, was reduced, breast cancer risk would fall.

Several studies have shown a protective effect of fruit and vegetable consumption (and in some studies, high fibre consumption) on the risk of breast cancer and have indicated that increase in consumption of these foods should be encouraged. One of these studies also suggested that high cereal fibre consumption should be encouraged. A large pooled analysis of a number of studies found that fruit and vegetable consumption was particularly protective of estrogen-negative breast cancers.

Height has been found to be associated with breast cancer risk in several studies, especially those evaluating the risk of breast cancer in pre-menopausal women, with the tallest women being at higher risk of breast cancer. Height, although largely related to genetic composition, is also related to adequate nutrition in childhood. It seems clear that the nutritionally deprived are at lower breast cancer risk. This may not be the entire explanation, however. For a woman to be tall, she has to continue growth through puberty, even after her periods have become established at menarche, and as we indicate below, age at menarche is nutritionally related. The effect of height is probably a complex relationship between continued production of growth hormone by the pituitary and production by the same endocrine organ of gonadotrophic hormones that increase the production of estrogens.

Obesity is clearly related to over-nutrition, and in its turn is found to be associated with breast cancer. Obese postmenopausal women have been found to produce estrogens within adipose tissue, and perhaps not surprisingly, obese postmenopausal women are at higher risk of breast cancer than women who have maintained a normal weight for their height. In premenopausal women, obesity is not associated with increased breast cancer risk, perhaps because the amount of estrogen produced by the adipose tissue in such women is relatively small compared to that produced by the ovaries themselves. However, premenopausal women who are extremely obese have suppressed ovarian function, and they have a reduced risk of breast cancer compared to women of normal weight.

REPRODUCTIVE BEHAVIOUR

Breast cancer largely only occurs in women who have, or have had, functioning ovaries for most of their lifetime. Indeed, breast cancer in males largely only occurs in those who for some reason or other, have had far greater exposure to female than male hormones, for example male transgenders who take estrogens.

In a woman, if ovarian function is lost early in life breast cancer will not occur. If a woman has her ovaries removed, or their function destroyed by radiation or high doses of chemotherapy given as treatment for other forms of cancer by age 40, her risk of breast cancer is reduced about threefold, and much more if the loss of ovarian function occurred before age 30.

These types of relationships are very direct and somewhat obvious. However, there are other indicators of ovarian function associated with reproductive behaviour that are related to the risk of breast cancer.

The earliest reproductive factor to operate in life is age at menarche. Women whose menarche occurred under the age of 12 have a risk of breast cancer about 50% greater than those whose menarche occurred over the age of 14, a relative risk of 1.5. This is a relatively weak risk factor for individual women, but very important internationally. The age menarche is established is related to nutrition, the poorer a girl's nutritional status, the later the age of menarche.

The average age at menarche is much older in poor developing countries than in the affluent West, and accounts for some of the international differences in incidence of breast cancer. Age at menarche has been declining in this century in the West and is beginning to decline in some Asian countries also. This accounts for some of the rising incidence of breast cancer in the world.

The latest reproductive risk factor to operate in life is age at menopause. Women with an age at menopause over the age of 50 have about 50% greater risk of breast cancer than women with menopause under the age of 50, again a relative risk of 1.5. Once again, this is a more important risk factor in comparisons between countries than between individual women within a country. Age at menopause is later in the West than in developing countries, and has been getting later in the West during this past century. Again, it seems to be nutritionally related and accounts for some of the international differences in breast cancer and the rising incidence of breast cancer in the West.

The direct relationship between age at menarche and menopause with duration of ovarian activity is easy to understand. Somewhat more difficult to grasp are two other risk factors related to reproductive behaviour: parity and age at first birth.

Two centuries ago in Italy it was recognized that nuns (nulliparous women) had about twice the risk of breast cancer compared to women who had had children. Looked at the other way round, the protective effect of parity is quite strong; women who have had four or more children have about half the risk of breast cancer than those who have had none.

There is also a strong effect of age at first birth. Women who have their first birth over the age of 30 have about three times the risk of breast cancer as women who have their first birth under the age of 20. Indeed, women who have their first birth over the age of 35 have greater risk of breast cancer than women who have no children at all. In practice, there is a strong relationship between age at first birth and number of children, in that women who have many children tend to start having children earlier in their life than women who have few. Although the effects of these two risk factors overlap, there is an independent effect of each.Prolonged lactation is protective for breast cancer. The effect is particularly seen in pre-menopausal women, and in women with prolonged lactation (more than five months). Indeed, if a woman delays her first birth beyond the age of 30, but ensures that the child is breast fed for at least five months, the increase in risk of breast cancer caused by her delayed first birth is nullified.

There is rather a complex relationship between pregnancy itself and risk of breast cancer. Women who have just completed a pregnancy are initially at higher risk of breast cancer than women who were not pregnant at the same age but who had the same number of previous children, or no previous children. This early effect of a completed pregnancy in increasing risk may account for the fact that women whose first pregnancy is over the age of 35 have a higher risk of breast cancer than women who have never had children. However, this effect of pregnancy in immediately increasing the risk of breast cancer (probably because of high estrogen levels at the last trimester of pregnancy) is soon replaced by the protective effects of pregnancy and lactation.

The effect of late age at first birth on increasing the risk of breast cancer is almost certainly not entirely due to hormone effects. It would seem that breast cells become less susceptible to the cancer-causing effects of chemicals and radiation after they have fully matured with the first completed pregnancy. The longer the time period between menarche and first completed pregnancy the longer they have had to encounter these cancer-causing substances. Delay in the maturation of breast cells, therefore, increases the time they are susceptible to the onset of the cancer-causing process and also increases the risk of breast cancer developing later.

Women with intact ovaries have three times the risk of breast cancer than women whose ovaries have been removed. In practice, this relationship varies with age. If a prepurbertal girl were to have her ovaries removed she would have hardly any risk of breast cancer at all. If the ovaries are removed before the age of 40 or receive irradiation such that they cease to function there is at least a one-third reduction in the risk of breast cancer. But if the ovaries are removed after menopause there is hardly any effect on the risk of breast cancer.

PHYSICAL ACTIVITY

Some years ago it was recognized that female athletes often developed anovular menstrual cycles, that is, their hormonal status was sufficiently affected by their activity so that they did not ovulate.

Whatever the mechanism for this effect, it is perhaps not surprising, from what we know about inhibition of ovarian activity and risk of breast cancer, that it was later demonstrated that female college athletes had a subsequently reduced risk of breast cancer.

What was more surprising is that studies of women who would not normally be regarded as athletes have found that those whose lifestyle involves at least moderate physical activity, including gardening, walking, etc., have a lower risk of breast cancer than sedentary women. Of course, women who are more active are likely to eat better, or perhaps more importantly, achieve a balance in their caloric intake with caloric output in activity and tend to avoid obesity. Whichever of these factors is dominant, it seems clear that physically active and nutritionally healthy women have a lower risk of breast cancer than their less healthy counterparts.

Genetic susceptibility

FAMILIAL CANCER SYNDROMES

For many years it has been recognized that breast cancer tended to occur more in some families than others and that when breast cancer did appear in some of these high risk families it often seemed to occur at a younger age, even in the 30s and, occasionally, 20s, and that in such families breast cancer seemed to occur more often in both breasts. Several investigators noted that when they evaluated the pedigrees of those rare families where breast cancer was extremely common, it tended to occur in a Mendelian dominant fashion—about half the women who were first-degree relatives—grandmother, mothers, daughters, sisters—eventually developed breast cancer. In such families they noted that the tendency to develop breast cancer could be transmitted by fathers as well as mothers and sometimes other cancers were more frequent also, especially ovarian cancer. It was also recognized that no more than 5% of the breast cancers that occurred had such strong family relationships, although there were some other families with less strong associations with breast cancer where the disease did seem to be more common than usual. It is now known that in these extremely high-risk for breast cancer families specific genes have changed, or in scientific parlance, mutated. We do not understand what causes the gene to mutate, but once a mutation in an important gene has occurred, the mutation is heritable—it is capable of being transmitted from parent to offspring. The two genes that are now recognized as being responsible for most heritable breast cancer are called BRCA1 and BRCA2. BRCA1 increases the risk of both breast cancer and ovarian cancer; BRCA2 largely increases the risk for breast cancer. It is suspected that there may be other breast cancer-related genes, but they have not been identified. Currently, it is believed that women who are carriers of BRCA1 have up to an 80% lifetime risk of breast cancer, with over half developing breast cancer by age 50, and about a 40% lifetime risk of ovarian cancer. Women who are carriers of BRCA2 have up to a 60% lifetime risk of breast cancer. Some researchers believe that these figures may be too high, as they are based on the first very high-risk families investigated; now some are finding carriers who seem to belong to families with lower risk. Whatever the risk eventually turns out to be, however, it is clearly very high compared to non-carriers of the genes.

Although most gene carriers are identified because they belong to a high-risk family, some have been found in a member of a family that, up until then, did not seem to be at high risk, probably because a new mutation had occurred.

Suspected causes of Breast Cancer

CHEMICAL AGENTS

A group of chemical substances that has attracted attention are the organochlorines. These are compounds that have entered our environment largely from the use of DDT and other chlorine-containing pesticides and herbicides. These substances tend to cumulate in the environment and get into our food chain. They are of particular interest with regard to breast cancer because some of them, or their metabolic products, have weak estrogenic activity and they are therefore termed xeno-estrogens. In the general environment there is good evidence that these compounds are associated with adverse effects on the fertility cycles of some animal species, having affected the thickness of eggshells of some birds associated with polluted lakes and rivers, as well as having affected male fertility by reducing spermatogenesis. Several studies have attempted to determine whether there was an association between the levels of such substances in body fat (organochlorines are lipophilic, or fat-seeking) and breast cancer, and some early studies suggested there was. Most recent studies of the level of these substances in the blood of women with breast cancer compared to those without have not shown an association, although there is some dispute about their interpretation and whether the study of levels of organochlorines in blood is optimal compared to studies in breast fat. Indeed, one study of organochlorines in breast fat in Canada has shown an association with breast cancer risk.

PHYSICAL AGENTS

Non-ionizing radiation from extremely low-frequency electric and magnetic fields (EMF) has been suspected as increasing the risk of breast cancer. Some studies of both women and men suggest that occupational exposure to high EMF levels may increase the risk of breast cancer, and there is some theoretical support for such an association. However, the data are not consistent and the mechanism of any increased risk has not been confirmed. For the majority of the population, any risk from EMF in increasing breast cancer risk is likely to be low.

DIET AND NUTRITION

Interest has been raised by the possibility that some aspects of the Japanese diet may be protective against breast cancer, as Japan is one of the low-incidence countries for breast cancer in the world. Soy may contain substances that could inhibit breast cancer development. Another potentially protective plant product is a component of flax. These substances are called phytoestrogens. It is postulated that they may interfere with normal or endogenous estrogen metabolism, thus reducing breast cancer risk.

REPRODUCTIVE BEHAVIOUR

There has been controversy over whether abortion, especially induced abortion, increases the risk of breast cancer. A series of studies have been contradictory, although a large study in the US designed specifically to evaluate this found that induced abortions had no effect on breast cancer risk.

SHIFT WORK

There is some evidence that women exposed to shift work at night, for example, nurses, have increased risk of breast cancer. Studies are ongoing to clarify this association.

Genetic susceptibility

FAMILIAL CANCER SYNDROMES

Some genes are suspected as being related to increased risk of breast cancer. The most frequent is probably the gene for ataxia telangiectasia (the AT gene). The mode of heritable transmission for the AT gene is different than for BRCA1 and BRCA2 in that it is what is called recessive—the gene has to be altered in both parents for one of their children (about one in four of them) to develop the condition called ataxia telangiectasia. This is a condition where the children from an early age are found to be extremely sensitive to light and other forms of radiation and liable to develop cancers (not breast cancer) at an early age. It is believed that women who are carriers of the gene who do not have clinical ataxia telangiectasia are at increased risk of breast cancer and also are sensitive to radiation. Some have suggested that as many as 15% of women in the population may be carriers of the AT gene, although the extent of their increased risk of breast cancer is not known.

Prevention

PRIMARY

Unfortunately, in spite of decades of study, we do not know all we would like to know about the causes of breast cancer; in particular, we don't know how precisely we can reduce the risk of breast cancer in individual women. However, most investigators now agree that the most important factors that can be influenced to reduce breast cancer risk are those associated with lifestyle, especially alcohol use, diet and physical activity, and smoking.

There are strong suspicions that the diet of girls and young women is as or more important than diet in adult life in reducing the risk of breast cancer. Girls and women of all ages should be encouraged to be physically active, to consume a diet with caloric content that matches their caloric output in terms of activity, to avoid excess fat consumption and where possible to substitute unsaturated fats for saturated fats, and to eat plenty of fresh fruits and vegetables as well as maintaining a normal weight. Provided that such a lifestyle begins sufficiently early in life, these women will have at least half the risk of breast cancer as their less health conscious colleagues, and, as we shall see later, will benefit by the reduction of other cancers as well. The benefits of such a comprehensive approach are not restricted to the development of breast cancer. In several studies it has now been demonstrated that obese women with breast cancer have a poorer survival than non-obese women. It has also recently been found in one study that women who had a lower fat diet before breast cancer diagnosis also had better survival than those with a higher fat intake. It is quite likely, therefore, that a healthy diet combined with physical activity and avoidance of obesity will benefit women who have been diagnosed with breast cancer.

Modification of reproductive behaviour is more difficult, although it seems clear that young women should be aware that if they postpone their first birth to beyond the age of 25 they will increase their risk of breast cancer, but they can reduce that risk if they breastfeed their infant for at least five months.

Secondary (early detection)

Screening for breast cancer using mammography has been believed to reduce breast cancer mortality by about 30% in women over the age of 50. However, a major study in Canada found that mammography had no effect in reducing breast cancer mortality, and it now seems likely that advances in breast cancer treatment have substantially reduced the benefit from mammography seen in studies conducted before improved treatment was available. There is some evidence that screening using physical examinations of the breast and breast self-examination are effective, and this may be particularly so in countries where at present breast cancer tends to be diagnosed at an advanced stage.

Tests for BRCA1 and BRCA2 are now available, but should only be used when there is reason to believe that there is a high risk of breast cancer in a woman's family. Their greatest value is to show that women in high-risk families who have not yet developed breast cancer are not gene carriers. Those found to be gene carriers have to make a series of difficult decisions. Do they want to rely on regular screening tests to find cancers early, recognizing that there can be no guarantee that the tests will find a cancer in a treatable stage? Are they prepared to undergo bilateral mastectomy with subsequent breast reconstruction, and, for BRCA1 carriers, bilateral oophorectomies (surgical excision of the ovaries) with subsequent estrogen replacement therapy? Even bilateral oophorectomies will not abolish the risk of developing ovarian cancer, as ovarian-like tissue with increased cancer risk can sometimes occur elsewhere in the abdominal cavity. There is evidence that women at increased risk of these heritable cancers will benefit by taking tamoxifen to prevent breast cancer, but with the disadvantage of an increased risk of endometrial cancer. Other hormonal agents are therefore being investigated, but so far none seem as effective as tamoxifen in reducing breast cancer risk.

Overall summary

In spite of an enormous number of studies, we are still not in the position to determine precisely why breast cancer occurs in each woman who is diagnosed with the disease. Indeed, many women who develop breast cancer seem to do so in spite of the absence of many or all of the risk factors discussed above.

However, we believe that most of the causes of breast cancer tend to operate relatively early in life. The lifestyle of young girls influences their future lifetime risk of breast cancer. Their activity and dietary lifestyle may be especially critical in this regard. It seems that mothers (and fathers) have a special obligation to help reduce the eventual risk of breast cancer in their daughters.

It is possible to make some estimates of the proportion of breast cancer caused by the various risk factors discussed in this chapter. Poor diet and over-nutrition resulting in obesity each contribute about 30%, as does late age at first birth, while lack of physical activity will contribute about 25%. Lack of breastfeeding and high alcohol consumption each contribute about 10%, while use of exogenous estrogens (hormone replacement therapy) and genetics each contribute 5%. Radiation may contribute another 1%. The figures are based on data from the Western world, but are rapidly becoming applicable in some of the developing countries as well.

Chapter 2

Lung Cancer

The term lung cancer is in many respects a misnomer, because the large majority of cancers that occur in the lung do so in the major air passages, the bronchi, which take air into and out of the lung. Cancers that arise in the bronchi are more correctly termed bronchial, or sometimes bronchogenic carcinomas, but the term lung cancer is in general use, and therefore I shall use it here. Cancers do appear to arise in the periphery of the lung, apparently among the air-containing tissue responsible for the processes of respiration, the absorption of oxygen, and the excretion of carbon dioxide. But even these cancers actually develop in the small bronchioles that arise from the air passages and link (like the branches of a tree) with the larger bronchi, and then the trachea (windpipe). So, although the appearance under the microscope of these peripheral cancers tends to be different from those arising from the large bronchi, they still are not derived from the tissue that is responsible for respiration. Cancers do not seem to arise from this tissue.

Lung cancers tend to occur as a mass that usually develops within the wall of a bronchus, but fairly rapidly spreads out into the surrounding lung when it becomes detectable on X-ray or CT scans. Some of the cancers in the largest bronchi spread into the centre of the chest and may involve vital structures in this area (the mediastinum). Because of the intimate relationship between lung tissue and blood vessels, lung cancers tend to spread fairly rapidly through the bloodstream, causing secondary deposits (metastases) in other organs including the brain and liver, and also other parts of the lung. The histology of lung cancers has been well studied; there are four major types and several minor, which tend to be grouped together. The major types are squamous-cell carcinoma, adenocarcinoma, small-cell carcinoma (with a variant oat-cell cancer included), and large-cell carcinoma. A form of adenocarcinoma that occurs in the periphery of the lung is called broncho-alveolar. Other specified carcinomas include adenoid cystic, mucoepidermoid, and large cell neuroendocrine carcinomas and carcinoid tumours. The proportion of adenocarcinomas is higher among females, and the proportion of squamous-cell tumours higher among males. There has been a tendency, largely for therapeutic purposes, to group all the non-small cell carcinomas into one group with this name.

There is some relationship between some of these histologic types and some of the causes of lung cancer, and where these have been studied I comment upon them in the relevant sections that follow.

The risk of lung cancer increases with age, although at older ages risk tends to decrease in most countries, probably because of a lower lifetime risk for older people who on average smoked less than younger generations. In the past, lung cancer occurred more frequently in men than in women, but more recently the risk has tended to become similar.

Lung cancer has been the most common cancer in the world for several decades. In 2012, there were an estimated 1.82 million cases in the world, representing 13% of all cancers. There are major differences between countries in the incidence and mortality from lung cancer, although these differences are narrowing as the tobacco epidemic engulfs the world.

Lung cancer is also the most common cause of death from cancer, with an estimated 1.59 million deaths in 2012 (19% of all cancer deaths).

The majority of cases of lung cancer (58%) now occur in developing countries. In men, lung cancer is the most common cancer (1.2 million cases worldwide, 15.3% of the total), with high rates in Central, Eastern and Southern Europe, North America, and Eastern Asia. In females, rates are generally lower, but worldwide, lung cancer is now the fourth most frequent cancer in women (583,100 cases or 7.8% of all cancers), and the second most common cause of death from cancer (491,000 deaths in 2012 or 13.8% of the total). The highest incidence is seen in North America, where lung cancer is now the second most frequent cancer in women and the number one cause of cancer deaths.Lung cancer was a rare disease in the 19th century and earlier, but, until recently, lung cancer incidence and mortality have been increasing in all countries of the world. The increase first began in several countries in men around the 1930s, and then, after two or three decades, began in women. However, in the last two decades, lung cancer has been declining in men in most Western countries. These trends are explicable by the changes in the amount of smoking in the population with the recognition that there is about a 30-year delay before the full effect of changes in smoking in the population are seen.

In general, the trends in incidence for females are upward, but beginning decades later than for men. The greatest increase in rates has occurred in the US and Canada. The rates are high in China (Shanghai) but there is insufficient data over time to determine the trend. Recently, there have been the beginnings of a decline in lung cancer incidence in females, noted first in the UK, and then in North America.

Mortality in general mirrors incidence. The UK has shown the greatest decline for men, and a beginning of a decline in women. Canada and the US are showing declines for men, but only recently for women.

The chance of survival from lung cancer is poor. Only about 15% of patients survive five years, although as for other sites of cancer, survival is better for those whose disease is diagnosed in relatively early stages. Survival is poorest in those with small-cell lung cancer, and somewhat better in those with other types.

In Canada, five-year survival relative to those of similar age and sex only increased from 14% in 1992-94 to 16% in 2005-7.

Lung cancer is believed to develop in the epithelium lining the bronchi, producing squamous-cell carcinoma and possibly other types as a result of changes in the epithelium, and adenocarcinoma probably develops from the glands that produce secretions or mucous in the bronchial wall. The earliest changes that can be detected with the microscope are the development of altered or metaplastic cells and proliferation of these cells (atypical hyperplasia). These changes can sometimes be detected by microscopic examination of sputum. A stage of carcinoma in situ (cancer cells entirely within the epithelium) probably occurs for many cancers, especially in the development of squamous-cell carcinoma, but is rarely detected unless a patient undergoes investigation with bronchoscopy (examination of the bronchi with a telescope, passed through the mouth and trachea). There is increasing interest in the possibility that finding such changes may enable those at high risk of lung cancer to be identified, with the possibility that medications might be prescribed that could prevent subsequent development of lung cancer, an approach called chemoprevention that is discussed in more detail later.

Proven causes of lung cancer

CHEMICAL AGENTS

The most important cause of lung cancer is cigarette smoking. Risk of lung cancer increases with amount smoked; both the amount smoked per day and the total duration of smoking are important, but duration has the greatest effect. Thus, someone who smokes 20 or more cigarettes a day will have about 20 times the risk of developing lung cancer than a lifelong non-smoker. However, a smoker of 20 cigarettes a day who smokes for only 10 years, will have about half the risk of someone who smokes 10 cigarettes a day for 20 years, even although the total cumulative amount smoked by these two people is the same.

The effect of duration is reflected in the effect of age at start of cigarette smoking. Someone who starts smoking under the age of 15 has about five times the risk of lung cancer than someone who starts smoking over the age of 25.

Once cigarette smoking stops, risk no longer increases, but it never returns to the risk of a non-smoker. If someone smokes for 20 years and then quits, his or her lifetime risk is only about a fifth of someone who smokes for 40 years. So the earlier that a smoker quits the habit in life, the lower his or her lifetime risk will be. There is hardly any increased lifetime risk of lung cancer for those who quit smoking before the age of 40. The type of cigarette smoked is also important. Per amount smoked, filter cigarettes induce less risk of lung cancer than non-filter cigarettes, and low-tar cigarettes less than high-tar. However, this does not necessarily translate into lower risk for those addicted to tobacco, as are the majority of long-term heavy smokers. Such a smoker smokes in order to maintain his or her blood nicotine level. You can guess the level a smoker needs to avoid withdrawal symptoms by the frequency he or she lights up!

In order to obtain the required amount of nicotine, an addicted smoker will usually draw more heavily on a low-tar, and therefore low-nicotine, cigarette than on a high-tar cigarette, thus effectively compensating for the lower nicotine, but at the same time absorbing a higher dose of tar and, therefore, more cancer-causing chemicals. There is no "safe", or even safer cigarette; the only way to avoid risk from smoking cigarettes is not to smoke them at all.

It used to be thought that women were at lower risk of developing lung cancer than men. However, this is now known to be incorrect. This misimpression was gained due to the fact that women started smoking heavily much more recently than men. It is now known that per amount smoked for an equivalent duration, the risk is the same in women as in men.

The type of tobacco smoked in some studies has been found to be important, the risk being higher for those who smoke cigarettes rather than pipes or cigars, as well as a higher risk for those who smoke "blond" or Virginia-type cigarettes than for those who smoke cigarettes containing black tobacco. However, this may be a function of the greater irritability of the smoke from pipes or cigars, producing less tendency to inhale than for cigarette smokers, or of black compared to blond tobacco. If a heavy cigarette smoker changes to pipe or cigar smoking and continues to inhale heavily there will be no reduction in risk.

Those who are heavily exposed to the smoke of others also seem to be at increased risk of lung cancer compared to non-smokers. This is called exposure to environmental tobacco smoke or "passive" smoking. This has been most easy to demonstrate for non-smoking women exposed to the cigarette smoke from husbands who were heavy smokers. A non-smoking woman exposed to about 20 cigarettes smoked by her partner per day in her presence for many years appears to have about twice the risk of lung cancer than a non-exposed non-smoker. On average, the increase in risk to non-smokers from environmental tobacco smoke in the home is about a 30% increase in risk. It has been more difficult to demonstrate a risk from environmental tobacco smoke in the occupational environment, but it is believed to be of a similar order to home exposure.

In some parts of the world tobacco is smoked in other forms than those familiar to people in the West. In India, for example, many people smoke bidis, a small cigarette-type device containing tobacco and wrapped in leaves. Studies in India have confirmed that bidi smoking causes lung cancer. It would seem that in whatever form tobacco is smoked, lung cancer risk is increased.

All histological types of lung cancer seem to have their risk increased by smoking. However, the risk is greatest for squamous- and small-cell carcinoma, and least for adenocarcinoma.

It is important to recognise that tobacco in any form is carcinogenic and if inhaled increases the risk of lung cancer. An example is the inhalation of smoke from water pipes (shishas or hookahs). It is often believed that harmful substances are reduced because the smoke bubbles through water. This has been shown not to be so. Indeed, the tobacco inhaled during one waterpipe session is equivalent to smoking many cigarettes. It is important that young people are made aware of this, and that anti-tobacco campaigns are extended to discourage water pipe use.

The effect of air pollution in increasing the risk of lung cancer has been difficult to study, as polluted areas are urban and industrial, and often cities have much higher proportions of smokers than rural areas. However, it is now agreed that external air pollution increases the risk of lung cancer by about 50% to as much as twofold in heavily polluted areas, clearly a much smaller effect than individual air pollution from active smoking.After smoking, exposure to carcinogens in the occupational environment is the second most important cause of lung cancer. There are a large number of such carcinogens, although as they are recognized steps are taken to reduce the level of exposure to workers, or even engineer the process so that workers are hardly ever exposed. As a result, this cause of lung cancer is becoming less important in the developed world over time. However, in developing countries, less care is often taken to reduce occupational exposure to carcinogens, and hence there is still likely to be substantial risk in many circumstances in such countries.

Among the chemical carcinogens occurring in the occupational environment that increase the risk of lung cancer are arsenic, (exposure in smelters and sometimes in drinking water), beryllium (refining, machining, and producing beryllium), bis (chloromethyl), ether (BCME) and chloromethyl methyl ether (CMME) (exposure in production of ion-exchange resins), cadmium, hexavalent chromium (exposure of chromate production workers and chromium platers), crystalline silica, some nickel salts (exposure of nickel refinery workers), and mustard gas (exposure of production workers in the past).

Some occupational exposure occurs to complex mixtures, many of which contain various polycyclic aromatic hydrocarbons, of which benzo-a-pyrene may be the most important (also found in tobacco smoke). Workers exposed to such mixtures include gas retort workers (in coal gasification and coke production), roofers and road workers (with exposure to bitumen and other coal-tar pitches), aluminium production workers (exposure to pitch volatiles), iron and steel foundry workers, workers exposed to welding (metal fumes may in part be responsible for the excess lung cancer risk in such workers), and transport and other workers exposed to diesel exhaust fumes.

Gold miners, especially in Canada and Australia, also have an increased risk of lung cancer. It seems unlikely that gold itself is the culprit, but rather, some other aspect of mining; this is discussed in relation to hard rock mining in general under suspected causes, below.

The classic example of a carcinogen encountered in the occupational environment that increases the risk of lung cancer is asbestos. There are different types of asbestos, chrysotile, crocidolite, and amosite being the commonest; all seem to increase the risk of lung cancer, although the risk from chrysotile is lower. Asbestos exposure occurs in asbestos mining, and in the production of asbestos-containing products (insulation materials, tiles, and brake linings, for example). Also, exposure due to use of some of these products, especially asbestos-containing insulation and other products in the construction industry, is also hazardous. The common feature of these exposures is circumstances where there is asbestos-containing dust—it is the inhalation of this dust into the lungs that results in the eventual occurrence of lung cancer. Once the asbestos has been stabilized in various products and used in circumstances where dust is not produced there seems to be little or no risk, as in asbestos-containing floor tiles and some asbestos cement products.

Concern over exposure of the general population to asbestos has led to its removal from buildings, especially schools, but also increasingly from other buildings where it had been used in the initial construction, usually for insulation purposes. Clearly, it is sensible to avoid exposure to friable asbestos where such exposure has been identified. But much of the removal has taken place under circumstances where exposure was minimal, and it is likely that the hazard to the workers removing asbestos was much greater than the miniscule hazard to those using the building had it been left alone.

PHYSICAL AGENTS

Ionizing radiation exposure that leads to increased risk of lung cancer occurs mainly in radium and uranium mining and milling. Although in such circumstances there is a form of radiation akin to X-rays (called gamma rays) that probably contributes to excess risk of lung cancer, the main culprit appears to be both alpha and beta radiation, the products of decay of radon. The extent of exposure in underground mines is dependent on the degree of ventilation. Once the risk was recognized, ventilation systems were improved, and the risk appears to have been reduced. It is of interest that although all histological types of lung cancer occur in excess in radiation-exposed workers, there seems to be greater risk for the development of small-cell lung cancer.

For both asbestos and ionizing radiation there is an interaction with smoking in that heavy exposure to both smoking and asbestos or radiation multiplies the risk of lung cancer. This seems to be a function of different stages of the carcinogenic process affected by the different carcinogens.

Radiation from radon decay products in homes built where granite or other ancient radon-containing rocks are close to the surface has been evaluated as a cause of lung cancer in a number of studies in Canada, Sweden, and parts of the US. Some of these studies were negative, but others showed small increases in risk compatible with low-dose exposures in uranium mining. The extent of ventilation in the home is clearly important, as well as whether radon decay product-emitting building materials were used in the construction of the homes.

DIET AND NUTRITION

There have been several studies evaluating the role of diet and nutrition in the occurrence of lung cancer. The one consistent finding has been that risk is higher in those with a low intake of fruits and vegetables than in those with a high intake. However, the precise protective factors in these plant foods are unknown.

Suspected causes

CHEMICAL AGENTS

A number of chemicals encountered in the occupational environment have been suspected of increasing the risk of lung cancer. Man-made mineral fibres are perhaps particularly important, as their use has now largely replaced that of asbestos. Most of them, including glasswool, rockwool, slagwool, and ceramic fibres have been classified as possibly carcinogenic to humans because they are suspected of increasing the risk of lung cancer. Glass fibres that are of much larger cross-sectional dimension than glasswool do not appear to increase risk, though there is some concern that certain forms of nano-fibres, which under the microscope appear similar to asbestos, may eventually be shown to increase the risk of lung cancer.

Hard rock mining in general, especially for iron ore, nickel, and tin, has been associated in some, but not all, studies with increase in risk of lung cancer. There is dispute as to whether the ore being mined or some other aspect of the mining environment is responsible, however. Radiation is a prime suspect, as it is in gold mining, but the studies that have been done of radiation levels in these mines have not always confirmed excess exposure. Elevated arsenic levels have been found in some mines, although for many the simple presence of excess dust, probably associated with excess silica exposure, seems to be the major correlate with risk.

Other suspect lung carcinogens include vinyl chloride and exposure to diesel engine exhaust.

DIET AND NUTRITION

Several dietary factors have been suspected as influencing the risk of lung cancer. High consumption of fats and/or dietary cholesterol has been associated with increased risk in some studies. An inverse association with high-fibre consumption has also been found, but it is not clear whether it is the fibre or some other constituent of fruits or vegetables that is protective.

In a large number of studies reduced risk of lung cancer was found for those that had a high consumption of beta-carotene-containing foods. This led to the evaluation of beta-carotene as a chemopreventive agent for lung cancer. In two such studies, those who were given high dose beta-carotene-containing pills and who continued to smoke showed an increased risk of lung cancer compared to controls given placebo pills. This unexpected finding led to a series of investigations that showed that the use of beta-carotene in high dosage interacted in some complex way to induce progression of the cancer in those who already had preclinical lung cancer.

GENETIC SUSCEPTIBILITY

There has been strong suspicion that there was an inherited basis for lung cancer. This was supported by studies that showed some increased risk of lung cancer in family members of lung cancer patients. However, no specific mode of genetic transmission was identified, and it is probable that at least part of the increased risk of family members is due to the tendency for relatives to adopt similar smoking habits. The feeling that something other than the play of chance determines which heavy smoker develops lung cancer and which does not persists, however. Part of this is a misconception relating to failure to understand the dominant effect of duration of smoking on risk of lung cancer. If humans lived for 200 years, nearly every smoker would die of lung cancer if they did not die first of another smoking-induced cause of death including other cancers, or heart or respiratory disease. In fact, we now know that at least half of heavy cigarette smokers die of smoking-induced diseases, losing on average 10 years of life as a result of their smoking.

Nevertheless, it is likely that there is multigenic susceptibility to lung cancer, related in part to the handling of carcinogens in tobacco and in part to the actual development of the cancer. A number of investigators are pursuing this possibility.

Unproven causes

CHRONIC INFECTIONS

Two diseases associated with chronic infection of the lungs have been associated with lung cancer in the past: chronic bronchitis and pulmonary tuberculosis. Chronic bronchitis is caused by tobacco smoking, and the association with lung cancer is probably due to this common cause. The relationship with tuberculosis is inverse, that is, lung cancer is less common in those with pulmonary tuberculosis than the general population, leading to the hypothesis that infection with tuberculosis was somehow protective, perhaps because of immunologic mechanisms. However, this association seems to be due to the lesser tendency for patients who develop tuberculosis to smoke than the general population.

NON-IONISING RADIATION

Extremely low-frequency electric and magnetic fields (EMF) have also been suspected as increasing the risk of lung cancer in some occupational and residential studies. Evidence of increased risk of lung cancer due to exposure to EMFs has been inconsistent, however.

Prevention

PRIMARY

The most important preventive action is not smoking, preferably not starting at all, but if smoking has begun, stopping as early in life as possible. As emphasised earlier, those who stop smoking by the age of 40 have hardly any increase in the lifetime risk of lung cancer. However, even stopping at older ages has a beneficial effect. Inhalation of smoke from waterpipes (shisha) should also be actively discouraged.

Other preventive actions include reducing exposure to occupational carcinogens and to environmental tobacco smoke, increasing intake of fruits and vegetables, and reduced exposure of the general population to radiation. Use of beta-carotene supplements in an endeavour to reduce risk of lung cancer is not recommended. Environmental contamination by asbestos dust remains a concern and measures to reduce asbestos exposure to all are very important.

SECONDARY (EARLY DETECTION)

It is possible to diagnose early lung cancer in those at high risk (such as heavy cigarette smokers) by using chest X-rays and sputum cytology. However, none of the studies of these screening tests conducted to date have shown any reduction in lung cancer mortality in those screened compared to those not screened. Recently, a large study in the US found that in heavy smokers annual screening with low-dose computerised tomography (CT) scans reduced lung cancer mortality. This study only used three annual screens and the comparison group was annual chest X-ray screening. Work is ongoing using mathematical modelling to evaluate the potential cost-effectiveness of low dose CT screening in heavy smokers, and several groups have advocated screening those considered to be at high risk of lung cancer. However, although it is sensible to be aware of the symptoms of lung cancer to prevent delay in diagnosis, screening of the general population for lung cancer is not recommended.

Overall summary

Lung cancer is unusual in relation to other cancers, in that a very high proportion of the cases that occur have a single known cause—tobacco smoking. In Western countries the proportion of cases attributable to smoking in men approximates to 90%, and in women in countries where the tobacco epidemic is well established, 80%.

All other causes are responsible for a relatively small proportion of lung cancers, for example, occupation 10% and radiation (especially radon in homes) 6-10%. The attributable fraction of lung cancer due to diesel exhaust fumes has been estimated at 1.5%. For many of these, the attribution overlaps with that of smoking, while the proportion attributable to low fruit and vegetable intake may be in the order of 15%. For women, the proportion of cases attributable to occupation is probably no more than 1% to 2%%.

Chapter 3

Mesothelioma

A mesothelioma is a cancer of the lining of the lungs (pleura), heart (pericardium), or of the abdominal cavity (peritoneum). About four times as many mesotheliomas occur in the pleura as in the peritoneum. They are rare in the pericardium.

Mesotheliomas have a very characteristic appearance under the microscope. They are composed of mesothelial lining tissue, and are non-epithelial in type, and therefore, although they are cancers, they are not carcinomas (a term restricted to cancers of epithelial tissue).

Mesotheliomas tend to occur largely at older ages, and, although rare, they are about five times as common in males than females.

In many countries (especially well documented in England, Wales, and Ontario, Canada) the incidence of mesotheliomas has been increasing over the last two to three decades, peak rates are not expected to be reached until about 2020.

Survival from mesothelioma is poor. The cancers are usually inoperable, and have extended widely within the pleura or peritoneum by the time they are detected.

Little is known of the natural history of mesotheliomas. There is some indication that pleural mesotheliomas develop in areas where the lining of the chest cavity has a scar, or plaque, formed of fibrous tissue.

Proven causes of mesotheliomas

PHYSICAL AGENTS

The principal cause of mesothelioma is occupational exposure to asbestos, particularly among shipyard workers, construction workers, asbestos miners, and workers exposed to asbestos dust in the manufacture of asbestos-containing textiles, insulation, asbestos board, brake linings, asbestos-cement pipes, and asbestos-containing tiles. All types of asbestos probably increase the risk of mesothelioma, although there is greater risk from crocidolite and amosite asbestos exposure than for exposure to crysotile (the type of asbestos mined in Quebec, Canada). Because of the paucity of cases arising in non-asbestos-exposed people, it is difficult to estimate precisely the extent of risk, but it is probably in the order of 15-fold or higher. Risk rises with the intensity of exposure to asbestos; most cases seem to arise after a very long latency period from first exposure. Pleural mesotheliomas can arise after relatively low exposure to asbestos; peritoneal mesotheliomas appear to require very heavy and prolonged exposure.

Asbestos is found in small quantities in the general environment, including drinking water, but mesotheliomas have not been conclusively associated with such exposures. However, mesotheliomas have been observed in individuals living in the neighbourhood of asbestos factories and mines and in people living with asbestos workers. In some countries it has been estimated that about one-third of the cases of mesothelioma arise from non-occupational exposure to asbestos.

Although in non-occupationally induced mesotheliomas the intensity of exposure to asbestos was generally less than in most occupationally induced cases, risk also rises with the intensity of exposure.

Other substances with fibres of similar size to asbestos may also induce mesotheliomas. This has been seen most conclusively in villagers living in one area of Turkey who are exposed to erionite, an asbestos-like mineral found in the soil and in the material from which houses in this area were built. High mortality from malignant mesothelioma, mainly of the pleura, was noted in three villages with erionite contamination among people who had lived in the villages since birth.

Unproven causes

CHEMICAL AGENTS

There is no relationship between tobacco smoking and the occurrence of mesothelioma.

PHYSICAL AGENTS

Exposure to man-made mineral fibres has so far not been shown to be associated with increased risk of mesothelioma.

Prevention

PRIMARY

The critical measure for prevention of mesothelioma is cessation of exposure to asbestos. In practice, in most countries, new asbestos exposure has largely been eliminated. However, asbestos is still present in old buildings, and appropriate care must be taken in their repair, reconstruction, and demolition. As indicated in the chapter on lung cancer, however, in the absence of exposure to friable asbestos, there may be more danger from programs to remove asbestos in stable situations than leaving it undisturbed.

SECONDARY (EARLY DETECTION)

There is no proven early detection maneuver for mesothelioma.

Although chemoprevention with beta-carotene was evaluated in asbestos-exposed workers in one study (and failed to exercise a preventive approach on the development of lung cancer), insufficient cases of mesothelioma occurred to evaluate chemoprevention for this disease. Given the increased incidence of lung cancer that occurred (as well as increase in mortality from cardiovascular disease), chemoprevention with beta-carotene cannot be recommended. No other agent is under consideration for chemoprevention of mesothelioma at present.

Overall summary

The majority of mesotheliomas are explained by exposure to asbestos, although cases have been reported where there was no history of occupational or environmental exposure to asbestos and no asbestos fibres were found in the patients' lungs after death.

Occupational exposure to asbestos in most countries accounts for at least 60% of cases and non-occupational exposure to asbestos no more than 10%. The remainder are unexplained, but it is likely that many of them may have occurred due to unrecognized or unrecalled asbestos exposure.

Chapter 4

Colorectal Cancer

The colon and rectum together form the large bowel or large intestine. The colon begins at the cecum, which is situated at the right side of the lower part of the abdomen, into which the small intestine empties. After the cecum, the colon becomes the ascending, transverse, and descending colon, followed by the sigmoid colon in the left lower part of the abdomen, the rectosigmoid at the junction of the colon and rectum, and finally the rectum, which opens to the exterior through the anus. In the colon the products of digestion from the small intestine are acted upon by bacteria, largely anaerobic bacteria (which metabolise substances in the absence of oxygen), and water is absorbed. The stool that forms is then passed to the rectum, which acts as a storage device until defecation occurs.

The anatomical divisions of the colon, and that between the colon and rectum are not precise and there can sometimes be confusion as to whether a cancer arises in the rectosigmoid area or the rectum itself. Further, the factors that increase the risk of these cancers often seem to be the same, or very similar, so the two sites are often considered together, a practice I shall largely continue here when the risk factors for these cancers are considered. When there is evidence suggesting different causes of cancers of the two sites I shall consider this.

Colorectal cancers are usually adenocarcinomas and they appear to arise from the glandular cells of the colon, with the initial changes probably occurring in folds, or crypts, of the epithelium. The basal cells of the crypts divide and the cells appear to move up to the surface where they are shed. These epithelial cells in the colon are among the most actively dividing in the body. It is this process of constant renewal or multiplication which appears to set the stage for cancer occurrence.

Colorectal cancers are usually classified as to the site in the colon where they arise (cecum, ascending colon, etc.). For some purposes they are considered as right-sided (cecum, ascending colon, right half of the transverse colon) and left-sided (left half of the transverse colon, descending colon, sigmoid, rectosigmoid) colon cancers, and sometimes the etiology of right- and left-sided colon cancers are compared. Cancers of the rectum are then considered left-sided.

In North America, colorectal cancer is the third commonest cancer in men and the second in women. It was estimated that in the world in 2012, 746,000 cases were diagnosed in men and 614,000 in women (53% in men and 55% in women in developed countries), while 694,000 deaths from the disease occurred in both sexes combined worldwide.

The incidence of cancers of the colon and rectum rise steeply with increasing age. Before the age of 45, both cancers are rare. For colon cancer, incidence is higher in men than women after the age of 50, but the difference is not large. For rectal cancer, however, incidence in men is nearly twice that of women.

As for most other cancers, there are major differences in the incidence and mortality of cancers of the colon and rectum worldwide, with the highest incidence in some of the developed countries. There are larger differences for incidence than mortality, with the region with the highest incidence (North America) having lower mortality than both northern and Western Europe and Australasia, regions with lower incidence. There is also a similar phenomenon for the comparison between southern and eastern Europe (including the former Soviet Union). Incidence had been rising but ceased to rise in the last two decades in Canada and the UK, but fell in Mumbai, India, which has low rates.

In contrast, mortality has in general been falling in most countries, except for Japan, where mortality was rising until about 1999. In Japan rising incidence and mortality is probably due to an increase in risk factors. Rising incidence and falling mortality could be due to early detection programs or changes in risk factors combined with improvements in therapy, with or without increasing efficiency in cancer registration. Falling incidence and mortality could be due to prevention programs. I shall discuss these different interpretations at the end of this chapter.

There are substantial differences in survival of colorectal cancer among world regions, with poorer survival in regions with relatively low incidence. Five-year survival is high in countries like the US (in the order of 60%), intermediate in Europe, (around 43%) and ranging between 29 and 37% in developing countries. Five-year relative survival (relative to the survival of similar people free of colorectal cancer) has been improving in Canada, from 56% in 1992-94 to 64% in 2005-07. The higher survival in North America may be a function of screening for colorectal cancer, as screening is advocated extensively there.

The colon and rectum is the classic site where a sequence of changes has been postulated in the development of cancer. The observed sequence probably starts with a focus of cellular change (atypia) in one of the crypts in the mucosa (epithelial lining) of the bowel. This focus enlarges and begins to intrude into the lumen (inside) of the bowel to become a potentially detectable small adenomatous polyp. There may be multiple foci of atypical crypts, and also multiple polyps formed. At first the epithelium of the polyps is almost indistinguishable from normal epithelium, but then changes occur in the direction of malignancy, initially with what is called low-grade dysplasia, then more severe high-grade dysplasia. Some of these dysplastic polyps become large polyps, which then change and become more disorganised—a stage often represented as villous change—and finally some change to cancer with invasion into the bowel wall.

It is known that in some families with inherited predisposition to colorectal cancer large numbers of adenomatous polyps can develop early in life (discussed further in the section on genetic susceptibility, below). Further, when autopsies are performed on adults who have died of other causes, the frequency of people found to have polyps in the large bowel increases with age, reaching about 40% in the elderly. This is much greater than the lifetime incidence of colorectal cancer, so it is clear that only a minority of polyps become cancerous, although the risk increases with increasing polyp size. Indeed, it is not certain that all cancers arise directly from polyps; some believe that polyps are a marker of risk and that cancers may arise from dysplastic change in the epithelium without necessarily going through a polyp phase.

However, it is clear that someone found to have polyps is at greater risk of developing colorectal cancer than someone free of polyps. Indeed, some proposals for screening for colorectal cancer have been based exclusively on methods to detect polyps, as discussed further in the section on secondary prevention (screening) below.

The adenoma-carcinoma sequence in colorectal cancer has now been linked to a series of specific molecular changes, a multistep process in which cells accumulate alterations in a sequence of genes that affect cell growth and differentiation, leading to the eventual production of a cancer. Several of these specific genetic changes have been characterised, with cancer occurring when the changes have cumulated to a sufficient extent for irreversible changes in cells to be produced.

Proven causes of colorectal cancer

CHEMICAL AGENTS

A prolonged history of tobacco smoking (more than 20 years) increases the risk of colon cancer, although at a much lower risk than for lung cancer. Smoking has also been associated in some studies (but not in others) with increased risk of adenomatous polyps.

PHYSICAL AGENTS

An increased risk of cancer of the colon was noted in survivors from the atomic bomb explosions in Japan, especially among those exposed at a young age. There was also an increased risk of rectal cancer among women who had received radiation treatment for cancer of the ovary. The colon and rectum, therefore, are regarded as radiosensitive sites.

However, colorectal cancer has not been noted to increase in workers occupationally exposed to ionising radiation, nor is the level of radiation encountered by the general public from radon in homes, medical exposures, or cosmic rays likely to be a cause of colon or rectal cancer.

CHRONIC INFECTIONS

Ulcerative colitis is a chronic inflammatory disease of the colon of unknown cause. Although secondary infection with intestinal microorganisms occurs, no primary infectious agent responsible for the development of ulcerative colitis has so far been identified. Some relief of symptoms (cramping pains, diarrhoea—sometimes with blood, loss of weight, anaemia) can be obtained by medical treatment, including steroids, but often surgical excision of the colon is performed. A major reason for this is that in sufferers from this condition, after many years, there is a substantially increased risk of colon cancer. The reason for this is uncertain, although the increased cellular division associated with the inflammatory process could be expected to promote carcinogenesis, and/or act as an inducing agent of progression for colon cancer.

DIET AND NUTRITION

A number of factors in diet affect the risk of colorectal cancer. Difficulty has arisen, however—as in all dietary studies in humans—in focusing on specific dietary causes of these cancers. The most consistency in various types of studies has been the protection offered by a fibre-rich diet, largely from vegetable consumption. Those who eat few or no vegetables on a regular basis are at increased risk of colorectal cancer compared to those who eat vegetables as a regular and important component of their daily diet.

It is unclear whether any specific vegetables are protective, or whether specific nutrients within vegetables are protective agents, although it is known that many constituents of vegetables are anti-carcinogenic in experimental animals, including allium-type vegetables such as onions and perhaps particularly garlic. Diets high in calcium, for example, dairy foods (especially low-fat), are also protective. There have been some studies that have suggested a protective effect of brassica vegetables (cabbage, cauliflower, Brussels sprouts) and other fibre-rich vegetables, as well as a few that are fibre-poor. The likely mechanisms for the protective effects of dietary fibre are discussed in the section on suspected causes below. Those studies that have examined the issue have found similar protective effects for both colon and rectal cancer.

It is now generally agreed that red meat consumption increases the risk of colorectal cancer. Meat in Western diets is a major source of animal fat, and there was some suspicion that this meat effect is an expression of such fat consumption, although the general view now is that it is a specific effect of some unknown component of meat. Some of the studies also found an association of increased risk of colorectal cancer with processed meat.

The majority of studies that have considered this have found a strong association between obesity and increased risk of colorectal cancer, especially abdominal fatness, as well as adult attained height, linked in some studies to over-nutrition.

ALCOHOL

There have been several studies that have evaluated the possible role of alcohol consumption and the development of colorectal cancer. The evidence is stronger for an association with rectal cancer than elsewhere in the large bowel. Beer consumption, mostly in males but also in one study in females, has been associated with a modest increase in risk, as have some other alcoholic beverages.

PHYSICAL ACTIVITY

There is strong evidence that exercise and physical activity at work and in leisure activities reduces the risk of colon cancer. Those who are physically active throughout life appear to have the greatest benefit, although recent physical activity also reduces risk of colon cancer to some extent.

The mechanism for this beneficial effect is unclear. It is possible that physical activity simply ensures proper use of energy-containing foods, possibly particularly dietary fat that otherwise would increase risk. Another hypothesis is that physical activity stimulates colon peristalsis (the intrinsic movements of the colon that promote passage of colonic contents), thereby decreasing the time that hazardous dietary factors remain in contact with the colonic mucosa. Yet another premise is that physical activity is associated with lower risk of obesity and together these reduce the risk of colon cancer through a hormonal mechanism related to avoiding resistance to insulin, the hormone responsible for carbohydrate metabolism, the deficiency of which causes diabetes.

Genetic susceptibility: Familial cancer syndromes

Familial adenomatosis polyposis (FAP), a syndrome that is inherited in a dominant fashion (directly from affected parent to child, with 50% of children affected by the condition), has now been linked to a specific gene on chromosome 5q. The syndrome is characterised by the development of multiple adenomatous polyps of the colon, sometimes amounting to several thousand. If no action is taken (colectomy is now almost universally performed on those with the syndrome), colon cancer almost inevitably supervenes.

Although affected individuals have this extremely high risk of developing colon cancer, the syndrome accounts for a very small proportion of colon cancers in the general population.

MULTIGENIC SUSCEPTIBILITY

The hereditary non-polyposis colorectal cancer syndrome (HNPCC) is much commoner than FAP, but difficult to distinguish from sporadic polyposis as there is no tendency toward extensive polyp formation. It is also inherited in a dominant fashion, therefore it will be suspected in a family with two or more individuals affected with colorectal cancer in more than one generation. It tends to have an earlier onset in life than sporadic (non-familial) colon cancer; right-sided colon cancers tend to predominate, and it is associated with an increased risk of other cancers, including endometrium, stomach, urinary tract and biliary system.

HNPCC is now recognised as being caused by germline mutations in DNA mismatch repair genes. A succession of specific mutations are involved and the syndrome has been associated with genomic instability and a form of genetic mutation called microsatellite instability, for which specific tests have been devised.

Suspected causes

OCCUPATION

Perhaps because of the frequency of colorectal cancer, occupational exposure to certain substances has often raised suspicions of causal associations. Perhaps the most consistent has been prolonged and heavy exposure to asbestos, which in several studies has shown an increased risk of colon and rectal cancer. Other exposures suspected include those in carpet making and the petroleum industry. However, the lack of consistency implies that these associations are probably not causal.

CHEMOPREVENTIVE DRUGS

Prolonged use of aspirin has been found to be associated with a reduced risk of colorectal cancer in a number of studies, although in several it was not possible to separate aspirin use from that of other analgesics. The one controlled trial that has evaluated aspirin use however, found no effect on colorectal cancer, although the duration of aspirin use (5 years) was relatively short. Nevertheless, aspirin has been associated with reduced risk of adenomatous polyps and in experimental animals there is sufficient evidence to indicate that aspirin reduces the incidence of colon cancer.

A similar anti-inflammatory drug, sulindac, has been found to reduce the frequency of polyp occurrence in patients with familial adenomatous polyposis. There is also sufficient evidence that sulindac reduces the incidence of colon cancer in experimental animals. There is some evidence that other anti-inflammatory drugs, such as piroxicam and indomethacin, may have similar effects.

Care must be taken over the possible use of these drugs because of the risk of toxicity, including bleeding from the gastro-intestinal tract.

CHRONIC INFECTIONS

Crohn's disease, a chronic inflammatory condition of the colon, can sometimes extend into the small intestine, with the formation of granulomatous areas with some resemblance to tuberculosis. However, in contrast to ulcerative colitis (discussed above), Crohn's disease does not have a strong association with cancer of the colon or rectum. Some studies have suggested a small increase in risk, but not to the same extent as for ulcerative colitis.

DIET AND NUTRITION

Total fat intake has been associated with colorectal cancer risk in both animal and human studies. The findings from the human studies have not been consistent, however, and interpretation of some of the earlier studies suggesting increased risk has been controversial.

There have been two major difficulties. First, in most Western populations in which the majority of studies have been done people tend to have fairly similar dietary patterns. It has often been difficult to distinguish the diet of individuals with precision and especially to separate off the effect of different sources of dietary energy or the protective effect of vegetables from the effect of nutrients such as fat, in increasing risk. Second, most of the studies suggesting increased risk due to fat were conducted by comparing the diet of cases with colorectal cancer with controls (case-control studies). The studies that assessed the diet in groups of individuals and related their risk of subsequent cancer occurrence to this information (prospective cohort studies) generally did not find an effect of fat in increasing risk.

The evidence for saturated or animal fat intake in increasing risk of colorectal cancer is somewhat better than that for total fat, although there is still a great deal of inconsistency. One of the large cohort studies did find evidence of increased risk, however, as did many of the case-control studies. The evidence is less extensive for rectal than colon cancer, but generally it is in the same direction.

Animal studies appear to be much more consistent in finding that dietary fat increases colon carcinogenesis. The mechanism may be the increase in excretion of bile acids in the gut, resulting from the digestive requirements for breakdown and absorption of fat, and consequent adverse effects on the epithelium of the bowel. Fat diets can lead to the destruction of the upper levels of the mucosa of the colon, with the consequent need for regeneration of the epithelium and the increased opportunity this provides for cellular aberrations to occur.

The overall conclusion appears to be that diets high in saturated or animal fat probably increase the risk of colorectal cancer.

Carbohydrates are an important source of energy, and in general have not been found to be associated with the risk of colorectal cancer. However, there have been some studies that have suggested a specific effect of sugar (particularly sucrose) in increasing risk.

Many studies in humans have found a protective effect of dietary fibre on colorectal cancer, particularly fibre from vegetables. The definition of fibre in diet is difficult, however, and several of the dietary studies in humans used information on the chemical composition of foods that did not allow estimates of total dietary fibre intake to be made. In animal studies, insoluble fibres such as wheat bran and cellulose are associated with protection against colorectal cancer, while some soluble fibres such as pectin are associated with increased incidence of colorectal cancer. One mechanism that has been postulated for a protective effect of dietary fibre on colorectal cancer is the increase in bulk of the stool caused by fibre, and the consequent dilution of any carcinogens that may be present. It is possible that much, if not all, of the protective effects of vegetables discussed above is due to dietary fibre. Yet, as indicated above, there are other components of vegetables that appear to be anticarcinogenic.

A large study of diet and cancer in 10 countries in Europe has shown a strong protective effect of high intake of dietary fibre. At the same time, a protective effect for the occurrence of polyps was found in a study in the US. The latter study appeared to contradict a trial of fibre intake conducted in the US, which showed no protection from fibre supplements. Possible explanations for this discrepancy include a short duration of follow-up in the trial and an effect of fibre upon the development of cancer in those with polyps, but not the development of the polyps themselves. Therefore, although most agree there is good evidence for a protective effect of fibre-containing foods on colorectal cancer, it is impossible to say at present that the protective effect is due to specific fibres per se.

Several micronutrients have been suspected as influencing the risk of colorectal cancer, especially the carotenoids, including beta-carotene and vitamin C. As for dietary fibre, estimates of consumption of such substances are based on intake of foods and there is insufficient evidence to separate off a protective effect from such substances from other protective factors in vegetables.

REPRODUCTIVE BEHAVIOUR

In several studies that have examined the issue, risk of colon cancer has been found to be higher in women of low parity than in women who have many children. This effect seems to be manifest largely for right-sided colon cancers. Two studies that specifically evaluated age at first birth found a greater effect for delayed first birth than low parity. The mechanism underlying these findings is unclear. There seems to be no direct relationship between use of specific hormones and risk of colon cancer. Rectal cancer seems to be uninfluenced by reproductive behaviour.

Prevention

PRIMARY

The most important factors that can be influenced by personal actions to reduce colorectal cancer risk are those associated with lifestyle, especially diet and physical activity.Actions taken in adult life are clearly beneficial, although it is possible that diet of children and adolescents is as important as diet in adult life in reducing the risk of colorectal cancer. Physical activity should be encouraged at all ages, both at work and in recreational life. Consumption of a diet rich in vegetables is clearly critical, together with consumption of cereals. Programs that encourage consumption of five or six vegetables a day should be supported. However, there is no justification for fibre supplements, unless prescribed for non-cancer medical reasons. Adequate fibre intake can be obtained through sufficient vegetable and cereal consumption. Encouraging low red meat and low saturated (animal) fat consumption is also important, together with a diet with calorie content that matches calorie output in terms of activity to maintain a normal weight.

Governments can encourage dietary modification by appropriate agricultural policies and sometimes importation policies. Subsidies that encourage red meat production and standards relating to meat that give higher quality grading to marbled (visible fat containing) meat should be discouraged. If subsidies are to be used in agriculture, they should encourage vegetable and cereal production.

Community planning to provide areas for recreational activity as well as office and occupational planning to reduce inactivity should also be encouraged.

It is clear that colorectal cancer incidence can change fairly rapidly (within 10-15 years), and thus preventive actions could be expected to have a fairly rapid impact. Given the attention that has been paid to diet, especially in relation to similar factors that increase cardiovascular disease risk, and the likely impact of such factors in explaining at least part of the reduction in cardiovascular disease mortality in many Western countries, it might be considered surprising that similar impacts have not been conclusively demonstrated for colorectal cancer. But perhaps they are—as indicated earlier, several Western countries are demonstrating a reduction in colorectal cancer mortality and a few also show signs of a downturn in incidence. The rising incidence seen earlier in some of these countries may have been artifacts associated with cancer registration, or screening.

SECONDARY (EARLY DETECTION)

Screening for colorectal cancer using the guiac faecal occult blood test was shown to reduce colorectal cancer mortality by approximately 20% in studies in the US and Europe. However, this benefit was achieved in the US study (investigation through endoscopy and X-rays) at fairly substantial cost in terms of false positives. The studies in Europe that used the test in a way that reduced the false positives achieved lower mortality reductions than in the US. In addition, the test has not shown to be sufficiently acceptable to be used by a high proportion of those at risk (over the age of 50).

A faecal immunochemical test, which is more sensitive for polyps and cancer than the guiac test, may be more effective and this has been evaluated in community studies. Hence, in many countries, screening for colorectal cancer using the guiac or immunochemical test is being introduced as public health policy. The diagnostic test recommended for those who screen positive to one of these tests is colonoscopy—the use of a tube introduced through the anus that can extend to the cecum. Non-availability of colonoscopy services has led to delays in introducing screening programs. In the US many advocate colonoscopy itself for screening, although because of its high cost and requirement for specialist gastroenterologists, this has not been introduced elsewhere.

There is now good evidence that screening using flexible sigmoidoscopy is also effective in reducing deaths from cancer in the sigmoid colon and rectum, an effect that may be due as much to the removal of polyps as to cancer detection. One or two such examinations, timed at the right age, might serve to identify a high-risk group of individuals who had already developed polyps for more intensive surveillance.

Overall summary

A large proportion (in the order of 50%) of colorectal cancers are explained by factors in the diet. The strongest evidence relates to fibre-rich vegetable consumption. High consumption of red meat and probably high saturated fat (animal) consumption are also causes. Low physical activity contributes to risk, as does obesity (accounting for approximately 20%), while genetic susceptibility explains perhaps 6% to 10% of colorectal cancers.

There is evidence that alcohol consumption increases the risk of rectal cancer, while occupational factors, especially severe exposure to asbestos, increases the risk of colon cancer.

Screening for colorectal cancer if high compliance is achieved could reduce incidence and mortality from the disease by 20% or more.

Chapter 5

Cervical Cancer

The cervix is the "neck" of the uterus. It is a muscular canal, lined internally with glandular epithelium, which merges into the lining of the uterine cavity. Externally it is lined with squamous epithelium, that is, epithelium that starts with a basal layer of cells and grows in successive layers and finally becomes thin and desquamates (or falls off) into the surroundings. This is similar to the skin, but thinner. This epithelium is continuous with (and identical to) the lining of the vagina.

At the place where the two types of epithelium meet there is a transition zone. In young women, the transition zone can be seen with the help of a small amount of magnification (usually by means of a device called the colposcope, which visualises the cervix through a speculum inserted into the vagina) just around the external opening or "os" of the cervical canal. In older women, the transition zone tends to be found just inside the cervical canal. It is in this transition zone that cancers of the cervix arise to spread and involve the external surface of the cervix, although occasionally, in older women, cancer may first arise within the cervical canal.

There are two main types of carcinomas of the cervix: squamous-cell and adenocarcinomas. As implied by their names, squamous-cell carcinoma arises from the transition zone in the cells adjacent to the squamous epithelium, while the adenocarcinomas tend to arise in the cervical canal and have a number of features similar to endometrial (uterine) cancers. Approximately 80% of invasive cervix cancers are squamous-cell.

Because the incidence of cancer of the cervix is so affected by screening, in most countries of the world with cancer registries, the incidence of the disease at different ages has been significantly affected by the screening programs. In one of the highest incidence areas in the world, Cali, Colombia, incidence is very high in middle age, but falls at the oldest ages. In most other areas, after reaching a maximum at about age 45, incidence remains at the same level throughout the rest of life. This is a different picture than most cancers, pointing to the importance of cervix cancer in middle-aged women as well as for older women; however, at younger ages (under the age of 30), cervix cancer in all areas of the world is rare.

The impact of screening on incidence by age has been well seen in Canada. In 1972-76, toward the beginning of the cervical cytology (Pap smear) screening programs in Canada, incidence peaked at age 70. By 2002-06 there had been a major impact, with substantial reductions from about the age of 30 in older women, but little at younger ages, when cancer of the cervix is rare. We believe that is due to the fact that for cervix cancer to occur in young women it must be rapidly progressive, and thus difficult to detect by screening.

There are very large differences in incidence of and mortality from cancer of the cervix worldwide. Cervix cancer is much commoner in developing than developed countries. Indeed, in 1990 it was the second commonest cancer of women worldwide, but the commonest in developing countries. It was estimated that in 1990, 98,000 cases of cervix cancer occurred in developed countries, but 371,000 in developing nations. With the increase in lung cancer in women worldwide, cervix cancer became the third commonest cancer in women, with 444,550 cases in 2012 in developing countries, and 83,000 in developed. The corresponding numbers of deaths from the disease were 230,150 and 35,500.

As already implied, incidence and mortality from cervical cancer have been much influenced by screening programs. This was well seen in the Nordic countries. All countries except Norway made a major investment in screening for cervical cancer from about the 1960s. All, except Norway, although starting at different levels of incidence, have shown a similar reduction in incidence. Norway only began to invest in cervix cancer screening once the discrepancy between their trends in incidence and that of its neighbours was demonstrated in the early 1980s, and only subsequent to that has any decline been seen. Trends in mortality are, in general, reflective of the changes in incidence. For some countries, an apparent increase in cervix cancer mortality in the 1950s was due to a tendency to certify deaths from cancer of the cervix to "uterus unspecified," and they were not then tabulated with cervix cancer deaths. In the UK there was a delayed reduction in death rates compared to Canada, Finland, and the US, similar to Norway, and for a similar reason as discussed above.

Survival from cancer of the cervix is closely associated with stage at diagnosis. Data from Sweden show that at the time of introduction of radium treatment for the disease in the early 1920s, the majority of cases were diagnosed in the advanced stages (stages III or IV), and survival within each stage was relatively low. With improvements in therapy, stage-specific survival improved, and there was some improvement in the proportion of cases diagnosed in the early stages following increased knowledge about the potential curability of the disease disseminated through public and professional education. After the introduction of screening these trends accelerated.

Most developed countries rapidly followed the example of Sweden. However, even now in most developing countries the majority of cases of cancer of the cervix are diagnosed in advanced stages. Recent data show that the overall five-year survival in North America is 68%, in Europe 61%, but in developing countries it largely ranges from 22% to 60% and in Uganda is as low as 13%. In Canada in 2005-7, the five-year survival relative to that expected from women of similar age was 72%.

The natural history of cervix cancer is understood better than many cancers because the cervix is so accessible to examination, and the cells that are exfoliated from the cervix can be examined under the microscope with the use of special stains. In practice, the epithelium of the cervix is scraped with a blunt instrument, or spatula, and the resulting collection of cells is spread (or "smeared") on a glass slide to be examined, or, more recently, the cells are suspended in a special fluid and the fluid examined on a slide, or through an automated reading method. This whole process is called cervical cytology, and the smears that are taken are often called "Pap" smears, named after the pathologist Georgios Papanicalou, who popularised the process.After the cancer-causing process has begun, changes begin to occur in the transition zone of the cervix, which are detectable on cytology. The earliest changes that can be detected go by a number of names: dysplasia, cervical intraepithelial neoplasia (CIN), or low-grade squamous intraepithelial lesion (LSIL). Dysplasia results in the nuclei of the cells undergoing changes that can be recognised; the cells, as they get nearer the surface, cease to be flat but retain much of their fullness, almost to the surface. Pathologists have distinguished various grades of dysplasia, called mild (CIN 1), moderate (CIN 2) and severe (CIN 3) to indicate their progress to lesions of greater severity. Severe dysplasia is followed by carcinoma in situ (CIS), a stage where the cells are indistinguishable from cancer cells and involve the full thickness of the epithelium, but where invasion into deeper tissues in the cervix has not yet occurred. Many cytopathologists now combine CIN2 and 3 with CIS as high grade intraepithelial lesions (HSIL). If progression continues, invasion will occur, and symptoms of the disease will be experienced by the woman (discharge, bleeding).

Regression (natural cure) is an important part of the natural history of cervix cancer. Indeed, regression is the rule for the earliest lesions (mild dysplasia, CIN 1 or LSIL). Recent studies have shown that moderate dysplasia (CIN 2) also more often regresses than progresses. Regression will also occur in a high proportion of cases of severe dysplasia and of carcinoma in situ (CIS). Even if progression occurs, it takes many years—8-15 years or more from the commencement of the process to the development of most invasive cancers. Therefore, it is important to avoid over-treating lesions discovered by cervical cytology. A standard recommendation of many authorities is not to attempt to treat cases of mild dysplasia (CIN 1 or LSIL), but to ensure that cytology is repeated after about six months. Only if the lesions progress cytologically, or persist after two to four smears, is excision recommended.

Proven causes of cancer of the cervix

CHRONIC INFECTIONS

Chronic infection with some types of the human papilloma virus (HPV) is now recognised as the necessary cause of cancer of the cervix. Many different types of HPV can be recognised, the principal oncogenic (cancer-causing) type is HPV-16, and the second HPV-18. Other HPV types are also causes of cervix cancer, particularly types 31 and 33.

Genital HPV infection has been found to be frequent in sexually active teenagers and young adults, both male and female. Risk of infection increases with each new sexual partner. Infection can persist in both the male and female, but in the majority appears to resolve spontaneously. Infection can be recognised by the cytological changes indicating the presence of the virus in cervical smears. Only a minority of women infected develop changes that progress to severe dysplasia and invasive cancer. In them, special tests usually reveal the persistence of the virus. This persistent behaviour appears to be restricted to the oncogenic (cancer-causing) types of virus. It is now recognised that cancer of the cervix cannot occur in the absence of infection with oncogenic HPV virus types.

CHEMICAL AGENTS

Several studies have shown increased risk for cancer of the cervix from cigarette smoking. The risk for cigarette smokers is about double that of non-smokers. A similar level of risk has been found for dysplasia and in situ cancer as for invasive cancer. It is now clear that smoking acts as a co-factor for HPV infection in increasing risk of the disease.

Oral contraceptives have also been shown in several studies to be associated with an increased risk of about 50% for cancer of the cervix.

REPRODUCTIVE BEHAVIOUR

Many of the reproductive risk factors for cancer of the cervix are the inverse of those for cancer of the breast. Thus, the disease is more frequent in married than single women, particularly in those first married at an early age, and increases in frequency with parity. The two major reproductive risk factors are young age at first coitus and multiple sexual partners, of which the latter is more important. However, the disease can occur in women who have had only one sexual partner, but then, it will be found that that partner has himself had multiple sexual partners. Thus, the disease is strongly associated with sexual activity in both males and females and this association is explained by the transmission to the woman of the necessary cause, an oncogenic type of HPV.

Suspected causes

PHYSICAL AGENTS

It is quite likely that the risk of cancer of the cervix is increased by ionising radiation. However, no human population is exposed to the level of radiation that would increase risk. The amount of radiation used to treat cancer of the cervix is so high that cells are killed, rather than cancer induced.

CHRONIC INFECTIONS

Several chronic infections that affect the cervix (other than infection with HPVs) have been associated with increased risk of the disease, especially infection with herpes simplex virus type 2. Much of the recent evidence has not supported infection with HSV 2 as a cause of cancer of the cervix. In particular, the virus does not seem to have cancer-causing potential. There is a possibility, however, that it may act as a co-factor for HPV infection in increasing risk of the disease.

DIET AND NUTRITION

There has been interest in the possibility that dietary carotenes, specifically beta-carotene, may be protective for cancer of the cervix. The evidence, however, is inconsistent; some studies showed a lower risk for those who consume more carotenes, others indicated no association. There have been similar findings for vitamin C consumption. However, those studies that showed a protective effect were unable to exclude the possibility that the vegetables and fruits from which the micronutrients are derived may themselves be protective.

REPRODUCTIVE BEHAVIOUR

As indicated above, high parity is a risk factor for cancer of the cervix. Given the strong correlation between sexual activity and parity, it is uncertain whether there is an independent role for parity over and above infection from oncogenic HPV viruses, although some studies in areas of high parity have suggested this. It is even possible that the trauma to the cervix associated with multiple births might stimulate cell division in the transition zone of the cervix that would act as a co-factor for HPV infection in causing the disease.

PHYSICAL ACTIVITY

Some studies have suggested that women who are more physically active have a lower risk of cancer of the cervix than those who are not. The association has been noted in both female athletes and for women with occupations that require physical activity. The studies that were done, however, were unable to evaluate the effect of other risk factors for the disease, and no biological mechanism that might explain a protective role of physical activity for cervix cancer has been proposed. Therefore, the possible beneficial effect of physical activity on risk of cervix cancer is as yet only suggestive and not certain.

GENETIC SUSCEPTIBILITY

Associations have been noted between the Human Leukocyte Antigen (HLA) haplotype (a genetically transmitted measure of immunity, evaluated in donors and possible recipients when tissue transplantation is considered) and cancer of the cervix. There is some evidence that certain HLA subtypes may be associated with HPV infection.

Unproven causes

CHEMICAL AGENTS

A popular hypothesis some years ago was that a carcinogen in smegma increased the risk of cancer of the cervix in the partners of uncircumcised men. The evidence linking circumcision to reduced risk of cervix cancer was inconsistent, however. Further, although there is clearly a male role in the etiology of the disease, it is now recognised to be because of the transmission from men to women of oncogenic types of HPV, not some carcinogen in smegma.

CHRONIC INFECTIONS

Of the HPV types recognised, two are often found in the cervix (sometimes with detectable changes on cervical cytology resembling dysplasia) where progression to cervix cancer does not occur. These are HPV types 6 and 11, the types of HPV that cause genital warts.

DIET AND NUTRITION

In general, studies that have evaluated the potential effect of dietary fat or meat intake in increasing the risk of cervix cancer have found no association. Similarly, although there has been considerable interest in the possibility that consumption of folic acid would reduce the risk of the disease, the conclusion now is that there is no such protective effect of this agent.

GENETIC SUSCEPTIBILITY

To date no familial cancer syndromes specifically affecting cancer of the cervix risk have been identified.

Prevention

PRIMARY

The most important preventive action would be to reduce the risk of infection with oncogenic HPV types. Until recently the only feasible approaches were those used for the reduction in the risk of sexually transmitted diseases; education of both young men and young women, use of condoms, reduction of promiscuity, and, in some cultures, changes to reduce the acceptability of males using prostitutes.

However, vaccines against HPV types 16 and 18 are now available and it is anticipated that vaccines that incorporate additional oncogenic types will be available within a few years. Programs to administer the available vaccines to girls age 11 or more (before sexual activity) are now being promoted in many countries. Some have advocated vaccination of similarly aged boys, as they are the transmitters of infection to girls. Vaccination of boys, however, seems unlikely to be cost-effective if adequate coverage of girls is achieved. It will be many years before such programs can have an important impact upon the incidence of the disease.

As means to prevent the disease there may be some additional roles for reducing parity, for promoting more fruit and vegetable intake, and for reducing smoking.

SECONDARY (EARLY DETECTION)

As indicated above, countries with successful cervical cytology screening programs can achieve at least a 60% reduction in incidence of cancer of the cervix, while theoretically, 90% reduction is possible with full compliance of those at risk and a high quality program.Unfortunately, it has been well documented that those at high risk of the disease are less likely to attend for screening than those at low risk, the latter tending to be the more health-conscious women. Organised programs, with full attention to all the details of recruitment and rescreening of at-risk women, adequate therapy of abnormalities, and high-quality screening tests are more efficient and less costly than programs that depend upon volunteer participation of women and ad hoc management of laboratories. Although the programs in Canada and the US have been successful, they have been largely based on annual screening and are extremely costly, whereas the organised program in Finland has achieved as great a reduction in incidence, with five-yearly screening at a far lower cost.

It is now recognized that screening does not need to start before age 25, and need be no more frequent than three yearly.

Low cost tests for HPV infection are anticipated soon. Because most HPV infection in younger women will spontaneously regress, such testing should not start before age 30. For older women, HPV testing may have a particular advantage, as those who test negative will not need to be re-screened for five or more years.

Few developing countries have yet been able to mount successful programs. Many have concentrated on younger women in maternal and child health services, leaving the older at-risk women unscreened and with little impact on the disease.

Overall summary

Cancer of the cervix has one necessary cause, infection with oncogenic types of HPVs.

However, the factors that cause HPV infection to persist, and the preclinical precursors to progress and fail to regress are largely unknown. The established cervix cancer control approach is cervical cytology screening from the age of 25 in an organised setting, but for older women this will probably be replaced by HPV testing. Organised programs must facilitate major efforts to ensure that all at-risk women are screened and that the program is administered with high-quality tests and treatment of abnormalities detected on screening. As HPV vaccination programs expand, there will need to be modifications of the screening offered to vaccinated women; HPV testing will then be of particular advantage.

Chapter 6

Endometrial (Uterine) Cancer

Endometrial cancer affects the epithelial lining of the uterine cavity—the endometrium. This is the tissue responsible for the cyclic changes in menstruation, which grows and thickens in preparation for implantation of the fertilised ovum and then sheds with bleeding if implantation does not occur.

The uterus is the site of the development of benign fibroid tumours (tumours of fibrous tissue). Occasionally, the muscular lining of the uterus itself will develop cancers; these are not epithelial tumours or carcinomas, but sarcomas. They are not endometrial cancers, and are of unknown cause. In the sections that follow I shall refer exclusively to endometrial carcinomas.

Nearly all endometrial cancers are adenocarcinomas. Around 3% are sarcomas, and less than 1% are squamous-cell cancers similar to those of the cervix.

In most countries, cancer of the uterus is rare at young ages and reaches a maximum incidence at about 60, then remains at the same level throughout the rest of life. This is a somewhat unusual age distribution for an epithelial tumour, but is rather similar to that for cancers of the cervix and ovary. It is believed to represent a lessening of impact of endogenous estrogens with menopause and a consequent effect on cancer risk.

There is wide variation in the incidence of cancer of the body of the uterus, with the highest rates in North America and Western Europe and the lowest in Africa and Asia. For mortality the highest rates are in Eastern Europe and South and Central America, including the Caribbean, although the lowest rates are still in Africa and Asia. Mortality in North America is, however, lower than all areas of Europe and Australasia.

The best survival for endometrial cancer is reported from North America and the worst in Africa and Asia. A special study of survival of uterine cancer patients in Europe revealed that overall survival, relative to that expected for individuals free of cancer, approximated to 60%, with little variation by country. As for other cancer sites, survival is influenced by stage at diagnosis, with survival for patients in advanced stages little better than 20%.

Hormones regulate the endometrium, with proliferation induced by estrogens, and inhibited by progestogens. Estrogens are secreted at the first part of the menstrual cycle by the ovaries, progesterone at the latter part of the cycle. This hormonal regulation of endometrial tissue is reflected in the evolution of endometrial cancer. The initial stage appears to be the occurrence of endometrial hyperplasia, often because of estrogen excess, which, if unchecked, can progress to early endometrial cancer. A stage of carcinoma in situ is also recognised.

Proven causes of endometrial cancer

CHEMICAL AGENTS

A number of studies have shown a consistent, strongly positive association between exposure to a number of estrogenic substances and risk of endometrial cancer, with increasing risk with both increasing doses of estrogen and increasing duration of use.

The most common such use is of non-contraceptive estrogens at menopause. These estrogen-induced cancers were often recognised promptly, in part because they induced unexpected bleeding and in part because women who take estrogens at menopause are usually under regular health care. Therefore, case fatality was low and seemed to have made little impact on trends in mortality from endometrial cancer in North America. Prescription of a progestogen at the same time as the estrogen seems to prevent the stimulatory effect of unopposed estrogens on the endometrium and therefore reduces the risk of such cancers occurring. However, this reduction is not complete, especially if estrogens alone have been used for some time.

Sequential oral contraceptives comprising an initial use of estrogen alone followed by a progestogen have also been shown to increase risk of endometrial cancer.In contrast to the effect of sequential oral contraceptives, combination oral contraceptives in which an estrogen is combined with a suitable dose of a progestogen reduce the risk of endometrial cancer. This reduction is in the order of 50% for usage over a period of at least five years.

Tamoxifen, a synthetic anti-estrogen used primarily for the treatment of breast cancer, has an estrogenic effect on the endometrium and therefore increases the risk of endometrial cancer. In clinical trials of tamoxifen as an adjuvant to prevent recurrence of breast cancer, the ratio of the rate of endometrial cancer in those taking tamoxifen was approximately four times the rate in those not taking tamoxifen.

DIET AND NUTRITION

There is a strong association between being overweight (especially with abdominal fatness) in both pre- and postmenopausal women and an increase in risk of endometrial cancer; obesity is causally associated with endometrial cancer in postmenopausal women. The mechanism is the secretion of estrogens by adipose tissue, thus excess weight induces endometrial cancer by a similar process as follows use of unopposed (by progestogens) estrogens. Obese premenopausal women do not seem to have elevated estrogen levels compared to non-obese women. A possible mechanism for the effect of obesity in increasing risk of endometrial cancer in premenopausal women is anovulation with reduced progesterone excretion.

PHYSICAL ACTIVITY

Physical activity is protective for endometrial cancer by virtue of its ability to reduce obesity (help maintain normal body weight by balancing energy intake with energy output).

REPRODUCTIVE BEHAVIOUR

Early age at menarche and late-age at menopause are associated with increased risk of endometrial cancer, presumably by a mechanism similar to that by which they increase the risk of breast cancer—by increasing the duration of ovarian activity and therefore the extent the endometrium is exposed to endogenous estrogens. Nulliparous women are also at increased risk; women who have had many children are at reduced risk, especially at young ages. There is no effect of age at first birth, however, in contrast to its important effect on breast cancer.

Genetic susceptibility

FAMILIAL CANCER SYNDROMES

The risk of endometrial cancer is greater for women with a family history of the disease. In patients with hereditary non-polyposis colorectal cancer (see chapter on colorectal cancer), the risk of endometrial cancer is also increased.

There are some other rare familial cancer syndromes in which risk of endometrial cancer is increased, often in association with increased risk of colon and breast cancer.

Suspected causes

CHEMICAL AGENTS

There is some evidence that smokers have a reduced risk of endometrial cancer. The mechanism may be a reduction in age of menopause in heavy smokers.

DIET AND NUTRITION

There is good, but not yet conclusive, evidence that diets high in saturated or animal fats increase the risk of endometrial cancer. In addition, diets high in fruits and vegetables appear to reduce risk.

Prevention

PRIMARY

The most important protective action against endometrial cancer is avoidance of over-nutrition and obesity. In addition, reduction in endometrial cancer will follow decrease in the use of unopposed estrogens at the time of menopause. If estrogens are deemed desirable, progestogen should be prescribed at the same time. Some care is required, however, in the use of progestogens, as it is possible that some of the other benefits of the use of estrogens at the time of menopause in terms of reduced risk of cardiovascular disease and reduction in osteoporosis will be negated by progestogen use.

The other protective action relates to the use of combination oral contraceptives.

SECONDARY (EARLY DETECTION)

Screening by means of endometrial sampling to detect the earliest stages of endometrial cancer in women at risk (obese women or those taking unopposed estrogens) has been advocated. However, no studies have been done that confirm that such screening reduces mortality from endometrial cancer, and no population-based screening programs for the disease are in place.

Overall summary

Obesity is the major risk factor for endometrial cancer, estimated to be responsible for 30% of cases; lack of use of combined oral contraceptives result in an additional 25%, non-contraceptive estrogen use and reproductive factors both 20%, and genetics 5%. These estimates have largely been derived from studies conducted in North America. Therefore, in countries where use of estrogens for the relief of symptoms at the time of menopause is uncommon, the effect of using estrogens will be much less, as it will also be if progestogens are prescribed at the same time. There is also likely to be overlap between the effect of some of these factors, so the fact that the percentages sum to 100% should not be taken to mean that we know all the causes of endometrial cancer. For example, the same women may use both combined oral contraceptives during their fertile period and non-contraceptive estrogens at the time of their menopause, with an overall reduced risk of endometrial cancer, especially if a progestogen was taken at the same time as the non-contraceptive estrogen.

Chapter 7

Cancer of the Ovaries

The ovaries are the paired organs in a woman's pelvis, attached by the fallopian tubes to the uterus, that are responsible for the production of eggs at the beginning of each menstrual cycle. The ovaries are also the main source of production in women of the female sex hormone estrogen. Present at birth, they develop and start functioning during puberty and atrophy after menopause when they largely cease functioning. Cancer may occur in the ovaries at any time during life, even in childhood. Usually just one ovary is affected by cancer. Ovarian-like tissue can sometimes be found elsewhere in the abdominal cavity, and ovarian cancer can occur in this tissue also. Although far less frequent than breast cancer, in many Western countries ovarian cancer is now the most important cause of death from gynaecological cancer, replacing cancer of the cervix from this position, largely because of the success of screening programs for cancer of the cervix.

Cancer develops in the ovaries as a mass, and the woman is initially free of symptoms. Symptoms tend to develop only when the cancer spreads beyond the ovary to involve other organs in the pelvis such as the intestine or bladder. Some cancers do not become symptomatic until the peritoneum lining the pelvis and abdomen is involved and fluid accumulates (ascites) to give rise to abdominal swelling, and eventually loss of weight. Hence, ovarian cancer tends to be fairly advanced when it is diagnosed.

Cancer of the ovaries is largely regarded as an epithelial carcinoma and is classified into four major types: serous, mucinous, endometroid, and clear-cell carcinomas. Adenocarcinomas, not otherwise specified, also occur together with germ-cell tumours and other specified types. Serous and mucinous carcinomas also include tumours of borderline malignancy (regarded as having low malignant potential). Patients with these tumours have a better prognosis than those not classed as borderline.Cancer of the ovaries has a somewhat unusual occurrence with age. Although rare, it occurs in children, especially germ-cell carcinomas. In adult life, when the epithelial carcinomas predominate (although the age of maximum incidence is around 75-79), incidence in middle ages is quite high. So, the increase in risk with increasing age is much more rapid than for many other cancers and the increase does not continue throughout life.

There is not as much variation in incidence of ovarian cancer internationally as for some other cancers, such as breast cancer. However, incidence is higher in Europe and North America than in South and Central America, Africa, and Asia. In these areas, mortality is much closer to incidence than elsewhere.

Apart from a rise in incidence in Japan, the incidence of cancer of the ovary has been stable in most countries over the period for which incidence data are available.

Trends in mortality from ovarian cancer show a slow rise in most countries over the 1955 to 1975 period, which continued in Japan, similar to the rise in incidence, but led to relative stability in the others. Mortality has fallen since about 1970 in North America, however, after a period of stability.

The rise of incidence and mortality in Japan is similar to the rise in breast cancer and probably reflects the "Westernisation" of that country. The recent fall in mortality but stability in incidence in North America probably reflects improvements in therapy.

Once ovarian cancer has spread beyond the ovary into the surrounding structures in the pelvis, survival is impaired. Survival is poor in Africa, Asia, and Central and South America. A special study in Europe in the 1990s found a five-year survival (relative to the survival expected in persons without cancer) of 30%. Survival is poorer at advanced ages. There is very little information on the natural history of ovarian cancer. One hypothesis is that this cancer is induced by errors in the process of repair of the surface of the ovary after ovulation. Thus any mechanism that reduced ovulation would reduce the risk of ovarian cancer. There is some support for this hypothesis in relation to the factors associated with ovulation as discussed below.

However, it is now believed that much, if not all, ovarian cancer initially develops not in the ovaries themselves, but in the fallopian tubes, which are in intimate relationship with the ovaries.

Proven causes of ovarian cancer

CHEMICAL AGENTS

Oral contraceptives, presumably because they inhibit ovarian function, reduce the risk of cancer of the ovaries. Risk declines with increased duration of use. Women who have used combined oral contraceptives for five or more years have about half the risk of cancer of the ovary than women who have never used oral contraceptives. Thus the absence of the use of combined oral contraceptives can be regarded as a cause of ovarian cancer.

DIET AND NUTRITION

A diet high in fat and low in plant foods increases the risk of ovarian cancer. There is also an association of adult attained height with ovarian cancer—the taller the woman, the greater the risk. The specific food groups or nutrients responsible are not known for certain.

REPRODUCTIVE BEHAVIOUR

There is a strong and consistent effect of parity in reducing the risk of ovarian cancer. The protective effect increases with increasing numbers of pregnancies, irrespective of outcome. Thus a woman who has had two pregnancies has about three quarters the risk of developing ovarian cancer of a nulliparous woman, and one who has had four pregnancies about half the risk. In this respect, ovarian cancer is very similar to breast cancer. However, the mechanism is probably reduced frequency of ovulation rather than reduced production of estrogen. There appears to be no independent effect of infertility as such.

Unlike breast cancer, there seems to be no independent effect of age at first birth, nor an effect of age of menarche or age at menopause in influencing risk of ovarian cancer.

GENETIC SUSCEPTIBILITY

For some time it was recognized that there were high-risk families for both breast and ovarian cancer. The gene that is now recognized as being responsible for heritable breast and ovarian cancer is called BRCA1. Risk of ovarian cancer does not seem to be increased in women who are carriers of the other breast cancer susceptibility gene, BRCA2. Currently, it is believed that women who are carriers of BRCA1 have about a 40% lifetime risk of ovarian cancer.

Suspected causes

CHEMICAL AGENTS

In one study a protective effect of regular use of the analgesic acetaminophen was found. In the same study aspirin use was associated with some reduction in risk, but it was not significant.

There is good evidence that smoking increases the risk of mucinous cancers of the ovary, but not other histological types.

In some studies there was a possible small effect of drugs taken for infertility in increasing the risk of ovarian cancer.

PHYSICAL AGENTS

Ionizing radiation appears to cause a reduction in risk immediately after irradiation, but after some years a small increase in risk. These effects have been shown in women who had survived for many years after irradiation for cancer of the cervix.

Two studies have suggested that women who dusted the perineum with talc had an increased risk of ovarian cancer. It was not known whether the talc contained asbestos (now very unlikely).

DIET AND NUTRITION

In several studies, women who consumed diets high in saturated fat had about a 50% increased risk of ovarian cancer compared to women who had low consumption. Women who had high intakes of vegetable fibre also showed reduced risk compared to those with low intakes. No consistent effect of micronutrients such as beta-carotene or other carotenes has been found.

In some studies, women who are obese have been found to show an increase in risk of ovarian cancer compared to women of normal weight, but this has not been a consistent effect.

REPRODUCTIVE BEHAVIOUR

Several studies have suggested a protective effect of hysterectomy on risk of ovarian cancer. This is believed to be independent of an effect of ovariectomy (removal of ovaries, which if bilateral would almost abolish the risk of ovarian cancer), but may be due to impaired ovarian function from interference with the blood supply of the ovaries.

A few studies have also suggested a protective effect of tubal ligation on risk of ovarian cancer.

Prevention

PRIMARY

The only proven protective factors for ovarian cancer are parity and use of oral contraceptives. Encouraging women to have children to prevent ovarian cancer would not currently be regarded as appropriate, although as for breast cancer, it seems important for women to be aware of the protective effect of parity in making their lifestyle decisions.

However, the protective effect of combined oral contraceptives on ovarian cancer should be borne in mind by women in making their contraceptive choices.

In addition, it seems very probable that a diet with reduced levels of saturated fat and high consumption of vegetables would also be protective.

The belief that ovarian cancer is induced in the fallopian tubes has led to the suggestion that women should have surgery to remove them. It is too early to tell whether this will become an established procedure.

SECONDARY (EARLY DETECTION)

There is no established early detection or screening test for ovarian cancer. Simple pelvic examination does not seem to be sufficient. Two screening tests have undergone evaluation: vaginal ultrasound to detect an ovarian mass, and a blood test for an antigen (CA 125), often found in excess in women with ovarian cancer. In a trial in the US, no effect of screening with transvaginal ultrasound or annual CA 125 blood tests on mortality from ovarian cancer was found.

Women found to be BRCA1 carriers cannot, on current evidence, rely on screening to protect them. Bilateral oophorectomies, with subsequent estrogen replacement therapy, are recommended for such women. However, even bilateral oophorectomies will not abolish the risk of developing ovarian cancer, as ovary-like tissue with increased cancer risk can sometimes occur elsewhere in the abdominal cavity.

Overall summary

Less is known about the causes of ovarian cancer than for some other cancers. Use of combination oral contraceptive is protective for cancers of the ovary—potentially 35% of cases could be prevented if all women used them. Nulliparity and diet probably each increase risk by 30% and genetics contributes about 5% of cases.

Chapter 8

Cancers of the Placenta

The placenta is the organ composed of both maternal and fetal tissue that ensures the transfer of nourishment from the mother to her developing infant during pregnancy. It is a very vascular organ, as it contains both maternal and fetal blood vessels to facilitate the transfer of nutrients. The cord linking the fetus to the placenta is composed of fetal tissue and blood vessels and arises from about the midpoint of the placenta.

The placenta develops at the very earliest stages of gestation, immediately after implantation of the fertilised ovum in the endometrial epithelium. It develops from the fetal side by the "invasion" of the endometrium and then the supporting fibrous and muscular tissue of the uterus by fetal tissue called "trophoblast." This trophoblastic tissue is able to grow into the uterus and may even spread into the bloodstream of the mother, but normal trophoblast disappears after the completion of pregnancy. The intermingled trophoblast and maternal tissue grows to become the placenta, an oval organ that at the end of pregnancy is about 12 cm long and 4 cm thick. It is discharged after parturition as the "afterbirth." Complete expulsion of the placenta is the rule, but rarely a placental residue remains in the uterine wall and cancer may develop in that remnant. This may also occur after a spontaneous abortion; indeed, it is possible that the development of an abnormality in the placenta is the reason for the miscarriage.

The main cancer that arises in the placenta goes by the name "choriocarcinoma" or "chorionepithelioma." This is a rapidly growing, highly malignant cancer, believed to be formed from fetal tissue in the placenta. "Chorion" is the name given to the epithelium lining the inside of the uterine cavity and covering the placenta itself, the outside layer of the extraembryonic membranes. Choriocarcinomas may arise after any type of pregnancy.

There are other tumours that can arise in the placenta. The most common is benign, and appears to develop from the tissue of a "failed" pregnancy. It is now believed to result from the fertilisation of an "empty" ovum (i.e., one without maternal chromosomes), as the chromosomes from this tissue are entirely paternal. This develops into a "hydatitiform mole," comprising collections of small cysts or grape-like lesions, which tend to be aborted and then the diagnosis is made. If a residue of a hydatitiform mole persists in the uterus, choriocarcinoma may supervene.

The other main tumour is called a placental type trophoblastic tumour. This is formed of tissue resembling normal trophoblast. It is usually benign, but occasionally highly malignant.

Placental cancers only occur during the fertile period of women. Therefore they tend only to occur between the ages of 20 and 45, with maximum incidence at age 30. They are still very rare at those ages, however.

The rarity of placental cancers makes it difficult to derive valid data, comparing rates in different countries. For example, for the period 2003-07, only 46 cases of placenta cancer were registered in Canada's national cancer registry, for a rate of 1 per million women/year. What data there are suggest stability in incidence and mortality.

Where modern chemotherapy is available, survival for cancers of the placenta is very good. Indeed, when diagnosed promptly these cancers are highly curable. The available data suggests that survival in the countries where incidence and mortality can be compared is in the order of only one death for every 30 new cases diagnosed.

CAUSES

Other than the association with pregnancy, nothing is known of the causation of placental cancers.

Prevention

EARLY DETECTION

A test for high levels of chorionic gonadotrophin (a hormone produced in excess by choriocarcinomas) is available. Therefore, with bleeding persisting after any type of pregnancy (whether to term or not) the test should be administered. Abnormally high levels of chorionic gonadotrophin will lead to other investigations and treatment if a cancer is diagnosed.

Overall summary

Placenta cancers are very rare and occur only in association with a pregnancy. With no known causes, prevention is not possible. However, with recognition of the possibility that a cancer may be present, early diagnosis is achievable, and a high cure rate follows modern chemotherapy.

Chapter 9

Vagina and Vulva Cancers

Anatomically contiguous, there are some features in common of cancers of these two sites, although in practice cancer of the upper vagina is more related to cancer of the cervix and cancer of the lower vagina to cancer of the vulva. The major site for vulvar cancer is the labia majora; for vagina cancer the primary site is the upper third and the posterior wall. Vaginal cancers may occur in women who have received surgery for cancer of the cervix. This seems to be an expression of a "field" effect—that is, the same causal factors acting on both the epithelium of the cervix and the upper part of the vagina.

The epithelial lining of the vagina and vulva is, in practice, similar to thin skin, so the dominant cancers of these organs are squamous-cell carcinomas.

Vagina and vulva cancers are largely diseases of older women. There is little difference in the incidence between Canada, the US, and England and Wales, but the rates in Japan in middle ages are substantially lower.

There are little differences between the incidence of these cancers in the West, but rates are lower in most parts of Asia, and probably most of Africa also. Throughout the period of recorded data rates are lowest in Japan, and to a lesser extent in other Asian populations.

In the US, five-year survival from cancer of the vulva relative to survival of women of similar age exceeds 70%, whereas for cancer of the vagina it is less than 50%. Similar survival rates for vaginal cancer have been reported from some developing countries of Asia. In Europe, relative survival from these two cancers considered together approximates to 50%; it is substantially lower in older women and higher in younger.

For both these cancers there is a phase of carcinoma in situ before invasion occurs. In some women, earlier (dysplastic) abnormalities have been found, analogous to those found on the uterine cervix.

Proven causes of vagina and vulva cancers

CHEMICAL AGENTS

A very rare form of vaginal cancer (vaginal adenocarcinoma) in young women and adolescents has been shown to be caused by the use of the synthetic estrogen, di-ethyl stilboestrol (DES), in an attempt to prevent threatened abortions in the mothers of these women.

PHYSICAL AGENTS

Ionizing radiation in the form of radiotherapy used for the treatment of cancer of the cervix has been shown to increase the subsequent risk of vaginal cancer.

CHRONIC INFECTIONS

Both vulvar and vaginal cancers are caused by chronic infection with oncogenic types of the human papilloma virus (HPV). For vaginal cancer, these are the same types that cause cancer of the cervix (16 and 18). For vulvar cancer, the same types have been associated, but so have a number of others. Benign condylomata of the vulva are generally caused by non-oncogenic (non-cancer-causing) HPV types and therefore they do not increase cancer risk.

Both cancers also seem to be increased in women with HIV infection.

Both cancers are more frequent in women of lower socio-economic status, although this may simply represent an increased exposure to oncogenic HPV types.

Suspected causes

CHEMICAL AGENTS

There is some suggestion that tobacco smoking may increase the risk of both these cancers.

DIET

There is some suggestion that both cancers are increased in frequency in obese women and in those with diabetes. This could possibly relate to some aspects of nutrition.

Unproven causes

REPRODUCTIVE BEHAVIOUR

There is no clear relationship between risk of these cancers and factors relative to reproductive behaviour.

Prevention

PRIMARY

Any measure that can reduce the risk of HPV infection (including vaccination) will reduce the risk of these cancers (see chapter on cancer of the cervix).

SECONDARY (EARLY DETECTION)

Women believed to be at risk for vaginal cancer because of prior treatment for cancer of the cervix should continue to receive regular cervical smears. The inspection of the genitalia and vagina that should accompany a cervical smear will also promote early detection of these cancers.

Overall summary

It is likely that at least 80% (or higher) of vagina and vulva cancer is caused by persistent infection with the relevant HPV types.

Chapter 10

Prostate Cancer

The prostate is the organ at the base of the bladder in males, responsible for producing much of the seminal fluid. It surrounds the urethra at its exit from the bladder and the spermatic ducts that carry sperm from the testes and seminal vesicles pass into the urethra through its base. Cancer can arise anywhere in the prostate, but most commonly arises in the periphery.

Most cancers of the prostate are adenocarcinomas that arise from the epithelial cells of the ducts or glands within the organ. Some cancers are transitional cell, similar in structure to those of the bladder and probably arise from the prostatic urethra. Squamous-cell tumours can occur, but they are very rare. Prostate cancers may occasionally be undifferentiated, showing little or no distinguishing features. Such cancers are usually highly malignant and have a poor prognosis. Cancer rarely arises from the fibrous tissue of the prostate; such non-epithelial cancers are termed sarcomas.

Prostate cancers are normally scored to indicate their degree of severity, or the likelihood that they will spread and potentially be fatal. A surgeon named Donald Gleason developed a common scoring system. The Gleason score is determined by an examination of a tissue sample under a microscope; a score of 7 or higher indicates a severe cancer, one of 4 or less an indolent cancer that is unlikely to progress.

Prostate cancer is largely a disease of old men. Internationally the highest rates are found in the US, while rates there are higher at every age in blacks compared to whites, and higher in the US and Canada than for the UK or Japan. Some of these differences could be due to different application of the PSA screening test for prostate cancer, discussed in more detail below.

Prostate cancer is the second most frequently diagnosed cancer of men in the world (estimated 1,111,700 new cases in 2012 or 15% of the total) and the fifth most common cancer overall. Nearly three-quarters of the registered cases occur in developed countries (758,740 cases). Incidence rates of prostate cancer vary by more than 25-fold worldwide and the highest rates are in Australia/New Zealand, Western and Northern Europe, and Northern America, largely because the practice of PSA testing and subsequent biopsy has become widespread in those regions. Incidence rates are relatively high in certain developing regions such as the Caribbean, South America, and Sub-Saharan Africa. The lowest incidence is in South-Central Asia.

With an estimated 307,470 deaths in 2012, prostate cancer is the sixth leading cause of death from cancer in men (6.6% of the total). There is less variation in mortality rates worldwide (10-fold) than is observed for incidence (25-fold). The number of deaths from prostate cancer is slightly less in developed than in developing regions. Mortality rates are generally high in predominantly black populations, very low in Asia, and intermediate in Europe and Oceania.

In countries like Canada the initial increase in incidence largely followed from increased use of diagnostic and screening tests, initially the tendency for trans-urethral resection of the prostate for urinary symptoms associated with an enlarged prostate, and later the increased use of a test for PSA screening.

The trend in mortality is not as dramatic. Nevertheless, there was an initial rise, followed by a fall. It is believed that the increase was due to what is called "sticking diagnosis," the likelihood that death will be attributed to a known malignancy in the patient without resorting to specific diagnostic tests. Some believe the fall in mortality is due to PSA screening, but the more likely explanation is prolongation of life from improved treatment for prostate cancer that will inevitably result in a reduction in death rates from the disease due to competing causes of mortality in the elderly.Survival from prostate cancer is poor in Africa and Asia and high in North America. There is a tendency for areas with lower incidence rates to have poorer survival. The explanation is probably the varying extent that countries are involved in active detection programs for the disease. In North America, where detection is active, incidence is high, mortality is moderate and survival is good. In Africa and Asia where there are no programs to try and detect the disease, mortality and incidence are close and survival is poor. Europe is intermediate, although detection programs are increasingly being introduced and the situation may change toward that of North America.

Survival varies by stage, as for most cancers. However, for prostate cancer the situation is complicated by a condition called latent prostate cancer, discussed further in the section that follows.

Enlargement of the prostate is common as men age. This is due to a condition called adenomatous hyperplasia, or benign prostatic hypertrophy. The enlargement can cause obstruction to the urethra, with difficulty in urination and eventually complete obstruction of the bladder requiring surgical treatment of the prostate. Adenomatous hyperplasia of the prostate is not a cancer precursor, although areas of cancer may develop within a prostate gland affected by adenomatous hyperplasia, and may be detected by chance when surgical treatment of the condition, required because of symptoms from the hyperplasia, results in part or all of the gland being resected.

At autopsy following death from other conditions, if the prostate is examined, small areas of cancer are often discovered. These completely symptom-free cancers that did not result in death are called latent prostate cancer. Latent prostate cancer is found increasingly frequently in older men. At the age of 80, 40% of men have latent prostate cancer. The frequency of this condition does not seem to vary as much internationally as does symptomatic prostate cancer.

It is suspected that all prostate cancers pass through a latent phase, and that all men who have normally functioning hormones are liable to develop prostate cancer. Indeed, it is possible that if men with latent prostate cancer found at autopsy had not died of another condition, symptomatic prostate cancer would have eventually developed in them. The cumulative risk of developing prostate cancer by the age of 80 is about 20% in US and among Canadian white males, but is less than 2% in Japanese males. Thus it would seem that about half of latent prostate cancers will progress to symptomatic cancers in men who survive to the age of 80 in Canada and the US, but a far lower proportion in Japan. Hence, for prevention of symptomatic prostate cancers, it is important to discover the factors that operate late in the natural history of the cancers and cause them to progress.

A marker of prostate cancer progression is a substance that can be detected in the blood of many men with prostate cancer, prostate-specific antigen or PSA, now also used for screening. (See section on secondary prevention below.)

In some men screened for prostate cancer, a possible precancerous condition, prostate intraepithelial neoplasia, or PIN, has been found. PIN can be confused with invasive cancer in the very small biopsies sometimes taken by needles when prostate cancer is suspected after screening with PSA. It is not certain that PIN is a precancerous condition; it may simply be a marker of increased risk of the development of cancer.

Proven causes of prostate cancer

Although a number of factors have been suspected of increasing the risk of prostate cancer (see below), no proven cause has yet been identified.

Suspected causes

CHEMICAL AGENTS

No clear occupational association for prostate cancer has emerged. In a few studies, it was suspected that exposure to cadmium in the occupational environment increased the risk of prostate cancer, and there has also been some indication that exposure to pesticides and herbicides through farming may increase the risk of the disease. In one large population-based study exposure to welding, synthetic fibres, some oils, pesticides, and aluminium compounds appeared to be associated with increased risk of prostate cancer.

PHYSICAL AGENTS

Ionising radiation probably increases the risk of prostate cancer, but there are no important groups at increased risk of the disease because of such exposure.

DIET AND NUTRITION

Associations of prostate cancer with energy intake, obesity, high fat intake and especially saturated fat intake have been noted in several, but not all studies. The associations have been more consistent when analyses have been restricted to patients with advanced prostate cancer, supporting an effect on the disease at the later stages of carcinogenesis. Increased risk has also been found in several studies for meat consumption. The possibility that high fat intake increases the risk of prostate cancer by influencing the later stages of carcinogenesis has been heightened by a study that showed that those who had a low fat intake had a better survival from prostate cancer than those with a high consumption of fat.

There is some evidence that high intakes of vegetables are protective for the disease. Specific factors in diet that have been evaluated include the carotenes, especially lycopene—found principally in tomatoes and tomato-based products—which has been found to exert a protective effect. However, for other carotenes, especially beta-carotene, the evidence has been more inconsistent, with some studies suggesting increased risk and some a protective effect. There are also suggestions that foods containing selenium are protective, while diets high in calcium increase risk.

In some studies, obesity has been associated with risk of prostate cancer.

REPRODUCTIVE BEHAVIOUR

There is weak evidence that some factors associated with sexual activity, including greater sexual activity when young and history of venereal disease, may increase the risk of prostate cancer. Vasectomy in young men has also been associated with the disease, although the evidence is inconsistent, and further study is necessary.

In one study an association has been found with levels in the serum of the male hormone testosterone and subsequent prostate cancer risk. The higher the level of testosterone found, the greater the risk of prostate cancer developing in the next 10 years.

PHYSICAL ACTIVITY

Although the majority of studies evaluating prostate cancer and physical activity have found a protective effect, some have found no effect, and two suggested increased risk associated with physical activity. Some of those studies that showed a protective effect found activity later in life to be protective.

Genetic susceptibility

FAMILIAL CANCER SYNDROMES

Men with a family history of prostate cancer in their fathers or brothers are at increased risk of the disease, and there are a few families where the risk is such that transmission of genetic susceptibility seems possible. There is also a possible association with BRCA1, the breast cancer susceptibility gene. So far, however, no gene that specifically increases the risk of prostate cancer has been identified, although several researchers are evaluating different candidate genes.

MULTIGENIC SUSCEPTIBILITY

Suggestions have been made that genes concerned with the metabolism of the male sex hormone testosterone or hormone precursors in the prostate may be associated with the risk of prostate cancer.

Unproven Causes

CHEMICAL AGENTS

Smoking has not been clearly associated with increased risk of prostate cancer, although some studies have suggested that mortality from the disease may be higher in smokers than non-smokers.

CHRONIC INFECTIONS

The prostate can be involved in inflammatory changes—prostatitis. However, prostatitis has not been associated with increased risk of prostate cancer.

DIET

An evaluation has been made as to whether alcohol consumption increases the risk of prostate cancer. No evidence has been found that moderate or light consumption of alcoholic beverages increases the risk of prostate cancer. There were insufficient studies of heavy drinkers to reach a resolution on the issue as to whether heavy alcoholic beverage consumption increased the risk of prostate cancer.

Prevention

PRIMARY

It is likely, but not certain, that reduction in dietary fat intake and obesity and increase in vegetable consumption would reduce the risk of development of prostate cancer. Given that this strategy is recommended for a number of cancers, as well as the reduction in cardiovascular disease, it should be regarded as a prudent strategy that is unlikely to have any adverse impact.

SECONDARY (EARLY DETECTION)

Screening with PSA has been advocated for prostate cancer, but evaluated with inconsistent results. A large study in several countries of Europe found a reduction in prostate cancer mortality with two to four yearly PSA tests in men age 54-69. However, there were inconsistencies in the countries participating in the findings and there appear to have been differences in the treatment offered to prostate cancer in the compared groups, which could explain the effect. In a study in the US, no benefit from PSA testing was found. PSA screening is not without adverse effects. The main difficulty is the possibility that screening will detect latent prostate cancers that are treated unnecessarily as the disease would not have caused death in the person's lifetime (i.e. over-diagnosis). Yet, many will experience some of the adverse effects of treatment, including impotence and incontinence. It has been calculated that the benefit from screening does not offset the adverse consequences on quality of life for those that receive treatment unnecessarily.

Overall summary

It is not possible to quantify the proportion of prostate cancers explained by the various risk factors discussed above because of lack of proof of causality. However, if dietary factors explain much of the variation in prostate cancer incidence and mortality (once the effect of early detection programs has been subtracted), at least 50% of prostate cancer in Western populations is potentially preventable.

Chapter 11

Penis Cancer

Cancers can occur on the penises of men, especially toward the glans. Penile cancers are almost invariably carcinomas of the external skin of the penis, and therefore over 90% of cases are squamous-celled carcinomas.

The incidence of penis cancer increases with advancing age and is largely a disease of older men.

The incidence of the disease is low almost everywhere, in the order of 1 per 100,000 men a year. The disease is known to be commoner in some parts of Africa and is rare in Jews in Israel. It is known to be higher in countries or areas with relatively low standards of living.

International mortality data are not readily available for this cancer.

In most registries rates have been low and constant. In Canada, between 1980 and 2007 incidence remained below 1 per 100,000. In the US a decline of 31% in age-standardized incidence of penis cancer was reported over the period 1973 to 1990. The rates for Jews in Israel have been the lowest throughout.

In the US the five-year survival relative to that for men of the same age has been reported to be in excess of 70%. In Europe the relative survival is similar, with little variation at different ages. In the few developing countries in Asia from which data are available survival approximates to 60%.

A carcinoma in situ phase is well recognised as part of the natural history of penis cancer. A condition named Bowen's disease, which is a scaly condition, occurring on various locations on the penis, but usually on the shaft, is a form of intraepidermal carcinoma in situ. Another pre-malignant condition that consists of red raised patches occurs on the glans and foreskin of the penis, named Erythroplasia of Queyrat, is also a form of carcinoma in situ. Both of these conditions appear to be true precursors of penis cancer.

Proven causes of cancer of the penis

CHEMICAL AGENTS

There is no question that the risk of penis cancer is lower in males who have been circumcised, especially if circumcision was performed in infancy or childhood. Further, risk is higher in those males who practice poor personal hygiene. This for some time was regarded as an indication of the carcinogenic effect of smegma, a wax-like substance that can accumulate beneath the foreskin in uncircumcised men. Indeed, some studies showed that it was possible to isolate carcinogens, especially nitrosamines, from smegma. It is still not clear if these observations support a direct carcinogenic action. More recently, other hypotheses on causation of cancer of the penis that do not involve chemical carcinogens have arisen, and these are discussed below.

CHRONIC INFECTIONS

The most favoured causal agent for penis cancer is infection with an oncogenic (cancer-causing) type of the human papilloma virus (HPV), the same viruses known to cause cancer of the cervix in women. International data reflects a positive correlation between mortality from cancer of the cervix in women and mortality from cancer of the penis in men. The wives of men who have had cancer of the penis are at increased risk for developing cancer of the cervix. Cancer of the penis is commoner among men who have a history of sexually transmitted diseases. Infection of the same HPV type in men and their female partners, and vice versa, has been demonstrated. The same oncogenic types of HPV viruses that cause cancer of the cervix (especially types 16 and 18) are associated with cancer of the penis in men.

The relationships between poor hygiene and lack of circumcision and cancer of the cervix can also be largely explained by HPV infection. In a special study in Spain, men who were circumcised seemed to be less likely to transfer HPV infection to their partners or receive infection from their partners. It was postulated that skin changes after circumcision result in greater resistance to infection with HPV.

Suspected causes

CHEMICAL AGENTS

Increased risk of cancer of the penis has been noted among smokers compared to non-smokers. However, as yet it is not known whether this is a direct causal relationship or whether the association with smoking with other unhealthy lifestyle actions results in the increased risk.

CHRONIC INFECTIONS

There is some evidence that risk of cancer of the penis is increased in states of immune system impairment, including AIDS. Again, this could be an indirect indication of increased susceptibility to HPV infection.

Prevention

PRIMARY

Primary prevention should principally concentrate on means to avoid HPV infection, including vaccination against relevant HPV types. Although the principal target group for HPV vaccines is adolescent girls, there is a rationale for vaccinating adolescent boys at the same time to reduce the possibility of infection being transmitted between men and women and also to provide protection against cancer of the penis in the men, although there is some controversy over its use. One other potential preventive action is circumcision.

SECONDARY (EARLY DETECTION)

Although there is no specific screening test, given the occurrence of precursor lesions, there is room to make young males aware of the need to seek medical attention promptly if they develop a lesion anywhere on their penis.

Overall summary

The proportion of penis cancers explained by infection with the relevant types of HPV exceeds 90%.

Chapter 12

Testis Cancer

The testis is the male reproductive organ responsible for the production of sperm. There are two testes, situated in an extensively folded sac of skin below the base of the penis (the scrotum). In an adult male, sperm are continuously produced in the testes, pass in the seminal fluid to the seminal vesicles attached to upper end of each testis, then into the vas deferens duct, which takes the seminal fluid through the prostate at the base of the bladder into the penis where it is discharged during ejaculation.

The majority of cancers of the testis are described as germ cell tumours, as they are believed to arise from the stem cells that divide to give rise to sperm. The commonest of such cancers are the seminomas (51%), followed by the teratomas (24%), the embryonal carcinomas (15%), and the choriocarcinomas (4%). The remainder are largely unspecified as to type. Rarely sarcomas arise from the fibrous tissue of the testis, but these only comprise 1% of testis cancers.

Testis cancer is largely a disease of younger men, with the major peak in incidence around the age of 30.

There are major differences in reported incidence of testis cancer, with the highest rates in Denmark, medium-high rates in Canada, the UK, and the US, and low rates in Japan. In Europe, the lowest rate is reported from Spain. There is nearly a fourfold range in incidence from the lowest to the highest rates. In other countries rates are lowest in Asia.

There is less variation in mortality than incidence, although the highest mortality (around 1990) was in Eastern Europe, even though other parts of Europe, North America, and Australasia had higher incidence.

Incidence almost invariably has been increasing, with Denmark holding its highest position throughout, followed by Canada and the UK. In Mumbai, India, there was no indication of an increase. In contrast, for most countries, mortality shows a somewhat abrupt decline, starting in the mid-1970s.

The contrasting trends of incidence and mortality for testis cancer are striking. The reduction in mortality is known to be due to the availability of new chemotherapy treatment in the 1970s, with a rapid improvement in survival of diagnosed cases. The reason for the increase in incidence is still unknown. This is further discussed below.

With the improvement in mortality, in spite of the increase in incidence, five-year survival from testis cancer in Europe and North America now exceeds 85%. The relatively sparse data available from the developing countries show a worse survival, approximating to 50% at five years in many areas.

All types of testis cancers are believed to arise from the same precursor, a form of carcinoma in situ without invasion. Differentiation then occurs in various directions and the specific histological types are formed. The stimuli responsible for these different types of differentiation are unknown, however.

Proven causes of testis cancer

CHEMICAL AGENTS

The synthetic estrogenic hormone diethyl stilboestrol (DES) was given to mothers in an endeavour to prevent spontaneous abortions in the 1960s. An increased risk of testis cancer in the sons of mothers who received DES for this reason has been found in several studies. Risk seems to be approximately doubled from the normal.

PHYSICAL AGENTS

A marked increased risk of testis cancer is found in young men with undescended testes. The increase in risk is about 20- to 40-fold. The testes normally descend from the abdominal cavity to their normal place in the scrotum about the seventh month of intrauterine life. There is some evidence that the frequency of occurrence of undescended testicles has been increasing in recent decades.

It is not clear why the increased risk occurs. The undescended testis is usually immature, but whether the hormonal factors responsible for the lack of descent are responsible for the malignant change, or the higher temperature encountered by the testis in its undescended resting place is responsible is also unclear.

Suspected causes

CHEMICAL AGENTS

In some studies, the use by mothers of exogenous estrogens other than DES during pregnancy has been suspected of increasing risk.

The association with estrogens and the increased incidence of testis cancer in most countries has led some to postulate that pollution of the environment with persistent organic chemicals, especially pesticides and herbicides as well as the polychlorobenzene products-PCBs (the organochlorines), may be responsible. This would link the increase in testis cancer with decline in male fertility, the reduction in sperm counts, and the estrogenization of many forms of wildlife. This is a controversial hypothesis that has been also linked with breast cancer but remains uncertain and which would be even more difficult to establish with the much rarer testis cancer.

Men in white-collar occupations seem to have about a twofold increased risk of testis cancer compared to blue-collar workers. The reason for this is unknown.

GENETIC SUSCEPTIBILITY

There have been suspicions, as yet unestablished, of some form of genetic susceptibility for testis cancer.

Unproven causes

PHYSICAL AGENTS

No link has been established between vasectomy and risk of testis cancer.

Prevention

PRIMARY

The only preventive actions known for testis cancer are the avoidance of prescription of estrogens to mothers during pregnancy and conduct of surgical operations to bring the testis down to the scrotum in those whose testes are undescended. It is unclear how effective the latter procedures are, as cancers have occurred in testes surgically placed in the scrotum.

SECONDARY (EARLY DETECTION)

Testis self-examination (TSE), to be performed by young men, has been advocated in the US. In general, promotion of TSE does not seem desirable, as incidence is low. However, awareness of the possibility of the development of testis cancer should be imparted to adolescent males to avoid delay in diagnosis if enlargement should be noticed.

Overall summary

Information is not available on the proportion of testis cancers explained by the various risk factors; for most cases, the exact cause remains in doubt.

Chapter 13

Urinary Bladder Cancer

The urinary bladder is situated in the pelvis. It receives urine from the kidneys via two tubes called ureters, and the urine leaves the bladder through the urethra. In the bladder, some concentration of urine occurs (i.e., water is absorbed), although the bladder largely acts as a storage device. If cancer develops in the bladder it occurs almost exclusively in the epithelial lining, which is three to six cells in thickness. This epithelium is structured to allow it to thin out as the bladder fills with urine.

As the epithelium of the ureters is similar to that of the bladder, if cancer develops in them, it is usually grouped with that of the bladder.

The epithelial lining of the bladder in which cancer develops is called "transitional" epithelium, hence the large majority of bladder cancers are transitional cell carcinomas. Some of these cancers are papillary in appearance (have fronds or papillae), which extend into the cavity of the bladder; these are called papillary transitional cell carcinomas. A small group (about 2%) of bladder cancers are adenocarcinomas.

Since many bladder tumours are papillary, showing neither invasion nor metastases, the diagnosis of carcinoma must depend on interpretation of cellular changes that indicate malignancy. These changes, called anaplasia, are subject to differences in interpretation according to the training and experience of the pathologist who examines them. The lack of standard criteria for the recognition of anaplasia in bladder tumours is reflected in great disparity in the incidence of papillomas and bladder cancers in various parts of the world, or even within the same country.

There has been a tendency, especially in North America, to regard papillomas without many distinguishing features of malignancy or anaplasia as being potentially malignant. This is because a significant proportion of apparently benign papillomas may be followed by carcinoma. There is no disagreement about the presence of a bladder cancer when it has infiltrated the bladder wall or caused metastases (spread to other organs). Carcinomas may be both infiltrating and papillary, papillary alone (when the diagnosis may be in doubt), or non-papillary and infiltrating.

There is also a form of superficial bladder cancer that may arise from cancer within the epithelium of the bladder—carcinoma in situ. Cells tend to be shed from such cancers, and they are often diagnosed by cytological examination of urine.

Squamous cancers of the bladder also occur. These are common in some parts of Africa and Asia where they are associated with an infestation of the bladder with a parasite (*Schistosoma haematobium*, described in more detail in the section on chronic infections, below). In Europe and North America, squamous-celled tumours of the bladder are uncommon.

A very small minority of cancers of the bladder arise in the wall of the bladder; these are then not carcinomas, but sarcomas.

The incidence of bladder cancer increases progressively with age, so that the disease is largely a disease of older men and women, although it can occur in middle age. Incidence is higher in men than in women. In the US incidence is higher in white men than in black males, but similar in women. Incidence is lower in India, but the increase in incidence with age is the same as for Canada, Sweden, the US, and the UK. Incidence is lower in both sexes in India.

With very few exceptions, the incidence of bladder cancer has been increasing for both males and females, although in some areas stability appears to have been reached and in Canada there has been a recent downturn in incidence in both males and females. Part of the increase seems to have been a diagnostic artifact, with the tendency for registration of papillomas as cancers that earlier would have been regarded as benign. However, some may reflect a true increase in incidence due to the impact of causative factors, especially smoking. (See below.)

Survival from bladder cancer is moderately good. For Canada the survival approximates to 77% for males and 76% for females; for Sweden the corresponding survival is 78% and 76%, respectively. For Canada, the most recent estimate of five-year survival relative to the expected survival of people of the same age and sex for both sexes combined was 72%.

Bladder cancer is believed to derive from a change in the epithelium, whereby the cells become anaplastic and grow either in the surface of the epithelium to develop into carcinoma in situ, or grow into the cavity of the bladder to become a detectable papilloma.

Changes of carcinoma in situ can be diagnosed if urine is examined cytologically, as cells exfoliate from the surface into the urine, retaining their characteristic malignant appearance. Superficial bladder cancer, a condition that can affect much of the epithelium of the bladder, is believed to arise from carcinoma in situ. If detected early, it is treatable by medication such as chemotherapeutic or immunogenic agents placed within the bladder.

Invasive (transitional cell) cancer can arise either from areas of superficial bladder cancer or from papillomas that develop more malignant (anaplastic) changes. Once it has invaded the bladder wall it tends to spread both within the bladder wall and into the surrounding structures of the pelvic cavity. If it is diagnosed at a stage where it is still within the structure of the bladder it can be treated by excision of the bladder (rarely in the case of small cancers by excision of part of the bladder). Once it has spread beyond the bladder, it is treatable only by extensive surgery or by radiotherapy.

Spread via metastases through the bloodstream is a late phenomenon in bladder cancer.

Proven causes of bladder cancer

CHEMICAL AGENTS

Tobacco smoking, particularly of cigarettes, is an important cause of bladder cancer. The relationships of risk with intensity and duration of smoking are similar to those of lung cancer, although the risks are lower. These relationships are seen in all countries where they have been studied, and in females as well as males. A few studies have evaluated the effect of different types of cigarettes. The effect of smoking filter cigarettes appears to be as great as the effect of non-filter. Risk diminishes in ex-smokers in comparison to continuing smokers within about five years of stopping smoking, but even after 20 years, does not completely return to normal. Risk of bladder cancer is lower in pipe and cigar smokers than in cigarette smokers, but is still much greater than in non-smokers.

Another important cause of bladder cancer is exposure to certain chemicals in the occupational environment. The aromatic amines used as intermediates in manufacturing dyes and pigments have been conclusively linked to bladder cancer risk in studies of workers in the dye and rubber industries, especially 2-naphthylamine, 4-Aminobiphenyl, and benzidine. This has led to their proscription in most countries. Other chemicals carcinogenic to the bladder include auramine and some chemicals related to the production of magenta. Working in the aluminium production industry has also been associated with increased risk of bladder cancer, possibly due to exposure to pitch volatiles.

PHYSICAL AGENTS

Though an uncommon cause of bladder cancer in the general population, radiation increased risk in the atomic bomb survivors and patients with ankylosing spondylitis who were treated by X-rays.

CHRONIC INFECTIONS

Schistosoma haematobium (a parasitic trematode, sometimes called a flatworm) infestation is a recognized cause of bladder cancer in Iraq, Egypt, and parts of Southeast Africa. In these areas, *S. haematobium* eggs are found in association with squamous-cell carcinomas, which rarely occur in the bladder in other countries. Chronic inflammation and infection related to the infestation may be the reason for the excess of bladder cancer, but the mechanism is not clear. The life cycle of *S. haematobium* is complex; eggs excreted from the bladder in land flooded with water (in Egypt from the Nile) infect snails where they grow and divide, then the parasites infect man through the skin and migrate to the bladder. Such infestation accounted for a high proportion of bladder cancer in these areas in the past, and also for relatively high rates of the disease. Although certainly still a cause, a recent study in Egypt suggests that smoking is now a far more important cause of the disease.

GENETIC SUSCEPTIBILITY

Bladder cancer has not been associated with familial cancer syndromes, but there is evidence that individuals can vary genetically in their metabolism of certain carcinogens that can affect the bladder. This is probably an example of multigenic susceptibility, likely to be evaluated in more detail in the future.

Suspected Causes

CHEMICAL AGENTS

Several chemicals are suspected as causing bladder cancer, including chemicals encountered in photography, benzidine-based dyes, and MOCA, a curing agent for plastics. In some studies exposure to dust and fumes was also associated with increased bladder cancer risk. Risk also seems to be increased with use of some paints. There has been much interest in the possibility that use of artificial sweeteners, especially saccharin and perhaps cyclamate, increases the risk of bladder cancer. The main evidence in support of this comes from animal studies, both those in which animals were administered saccharin over more than one generation, and those in which saccharin and cyclamate were administered in conjunction with low doses of known bladder carcinogens. The human evidence has been somewhat contradictory, with most studies showing little or no increase in risk, but some showing increase restricted to certain subgroups, such as non-smokers.

PHYSICAL AGENTS

In experimental animals, bladder stones clearly increase the risk of bladder cancer. In humans, bladder stones rarely occur, and even if they do are treated. So this possible cause of the past is, at least in developed countries, no longer a potential cause of bladder cancer.

CHRONIC INFECTIONS

Some studies have suggested that chronic urinary infections (cystitis) can increase the risk of bladder cancer. Again, with the availability of antibiotics or other agents to treat bladder infections, chronic infections are now rare and unlikely to be responsible for much in the way of bladder cancer.

DIET AND NUTRITION

By far the most consistent evidence on the effect of diet on risk of bladder cancer relates to fruit and vegetable intake, which, in the majority of studies that evaluated diet, was protective for bladder cancer. Earlier studies tended to evaluate micronutrients derived from vegetables or fruit, such as beta-carotene or vitamin A. The majority of such studies found a protective effect of high intake of beta-carotene, but not of preformed vitamin A (from animal sources). However, it cannot be concluded that beta-carotene per se is the protective factor; it is probable that some other factor in vegetables or fruits is responsible for the protective effect.Some studies have suggested that intake of dietary fat may increase the risk of bladder cancer, and one found a strong effect of dietary cholesterol in increasing risk. If fruits and vegetables reduce the risk of bladder cancer, there must be other factors that increase risk and dietary fat and/or cholesterol intake are potential candidates, but so far the evidence to support intake of fat as increasing risk is not strong.

Coffee has been investigated in a number of studies as increasing the risk of bladder cancer. Part of the difficulty in evaluating coffee is that high intake is positively correlated with cigarette smoking, the main established cause of bladder cancer. Several studies did not adequately control for the effects of smoking, but in those that did an apparent effect of coffee intake in increasing risk was attenuated.

Alcohol is established as not influencing bladder cancer risk. Bladder cancer has also not been associated with reproductive activity.

Prevention

PRIMARY PREVENTION

The most important preventive activity for bladder cancer is to reduce smoking, especially of cigarettes. The main benefit will come from prevention of smoking onset in childhood, but substantial benefit can be expected from effective smoking cessation programs in adults, especially if smokers can be persuaded to stop relatively early in life.

The second important preventive activity is to reduce occupational exposure to known bladder carcinogens. Much has been accomplished in this respect in developed countries, but in some instances the production of known bladder carcinogens has been transferred from developed to developing countries, so the world has not yet been cleared from the hazard of occupationally induced bladder cancer.A third preventive activity that is likely to reduce bladder cancer risk is dietary modification, especially increase in vegetable and fruit intake. Although the primary reason to promote dietary modification for cancer control is not bladder cancer, it is probable that bladder cancer risk will be reduced by programs that promote increased vegetable and fruit intake for prevention of other cancers, such as cancer of the colon and rectum.

In parts of Africa and the Middle East, reinforcing control programs to reduce human infestation with *Schisosoma haematobium* will reduce bladder cancer in those areas. Although in urban areas in Egypt tobacco smoking is a much more important cause of bladder cancer than the consequences of schistosomiasis, in rural areas that may not be the case. There is a potential conflict between the economic benefits derived from irrigation schemes that may lead to the maintenance of the snail habitats of the secondary host of the schistosomes, and prevention of bladder cancer. However, the mechanisms for control are available; educational programs to avoid walking in water unprotected as well as programs that distribute the necessary molluscides (drugs that kill snails) are required to reduce the hazard.

SECONDARY (EARLY DETECTION)

Urinary cytology as a screen for bladder cancer has been employed in some industrial populations at increased risk for bladder cancer and investigated in one study in Egypt. A major difficulty is that the test is most sensitive for in situ cancer of the bladder, and not for invasive cancer. As an individual secondary prevention activity, urinary cytology therefore has and can have little impact. It is of more value as a means to identify a high-risk group upon whom primary preventive activities should be concentrated.

Overall summary

Approximately 60% of bladder cancers are caused by tobacco smoking, and 20% from occupational factors. Poor diet may cause 20% of cases, although the evidence for diet as a cause is not strong.

Schistosomiasis probably causes about 15% of cases in the world, for example in Egypt, although in a recent investigation there the proportion of bladder cancer attributed to tobacco was 75%. Indeed, it is probable that everywhere the proportion of bladder cancer attributable to tobacco is increasing while the proportion attributable to occupational causes is becoming much less. It is apparent, therefore, that bladder cancer is largely a preventable disease.

Chapter 14

Kidney Cancers

The kidneys are paired organs lying behind the peritoneum (the lining of the abdominal cavity) under the diaphragm. They are responsible for excreting waste products from the blood into the urine, which collects in a sac (the renal pelvis) on the inside of each kidney then passes down to the bladder through a narrow muscular tube (the ureter). The kidneys have a good blood supply from the renal artery that branches from the main blood-carrying artery coming from the heart into the abdomen (the aorta), and the blood drains back in the renal vein to the large vein going back to the heart (the inferior vena cava). They are relatively insensitive organs, but if a stone occludes the upper part of the ureter severe pain will be felt in the back on the same side (renal colic).

There are two different types of kidney cancer, depending on whether they arise in the body of the kidney (renal cell carcinoma) or in the renal pelvis. Cancers of the renal pelvis have the same histological appearance as cancers of the ureter and bladder and are called transitional cell or sometimes, especially in the renal pelvis, squamous-cell cancers occur. In children, a special form of kidney cancer occurs, which is believed to arise from primitive (embryonal) cells; this is called a nephroblastoma, or Wilm's tumour. Of all kidney cancers 88% are cancers of the body of the kidney in adults, 9% renal pelvis cancers, and 2% Wilm's tumours.

In most cancer registries and vital statistics systems cancers of the body of the kidney and of the renal pelvis are grouped together, sometimes with the uncommon cancers of the ureters. Thus, the section below relates to this grouping. Most of what follows relates to renal cell carcinoma; where there are differences with renal pelvis cancers these will be described.

Kidney cancer is largely a disease of older people, although there is a small rise in incidence at the youngest ages due to Wilm's tumour. It is similar in incidence in Canada and the US, but lower in the UK and Japan, in all about twice as high in males as in females.

There are large differences in incidence of kidney cancer worldwide, with the highest rates in North America and Western Europe and the lowest in Africa and Asia. Mortality differences are less, with higher mortality in Western, Eastern, and Northern Europe than in North America. Everywhere rates are higher in males than females.

Almost universally, in the last two decades there has been an increase in incidence of kidney cancer, both in males and females, although the increase is least in low-incidence areas such as India (Mumbai). For mortality there has been relative stability in Canada, the US, and the UK in both males and females, but in Japan, mortality in males increased substantially.

Survival from kidney cancer is much better in developed than in developing countries, with survival as low as 10% in males and 17% in females at five years in one area of Thailand, while in Shanghai it was as high as 40% in males, and 45% in females. These rates mirror those reported from several registries in Europe, where the five-year survival can be 40% or more. In Canada, there has been an increase in five-year survival relative to people of the same age and sex from 60% in 1992-94 to 67% in 2005-07.

As the kidney is relatively inaccessible, not a great deal is known about its natural history. There is no clearly recognised renal cell cancer precursor. However, some small cancers of the kidney are found accidentally, as a result of an X-ray or CT scan of the abdomen. Although most of these are removed, in some patients they have been simply observed, and appear not to grow. Indeed, some cases have been documented that are known to have been present without causing symptoms for 20 years or more.

Proven causes of kidney cancer

CHEMICAL AGENTS

The most important known cause of kidney cancer is tobacco smoking. The risk of renal cell carcinoma is increased about two- to threefold by cigarette smoking. However, the rarer pelvic (transitional cell) cancers are increased to a much greater extent by smoking. Indeed, the majority of these cancers are due to this cause, which is not the case for the commoner renal cell cancers of the body of the kidney. It seems likely that much of the increase in both incidence and mortality from kidney cancer in many countries is due to smoking.

The other known cause of renal pelvis cancer is chronic use of phenacetin-type analgesics over many years; the greater the dose, the greater the risk.

PHYSICAL AGENTS

Ionizing radiation has been found to increase the risk of kidney cancer in some studies of the medical use of radiation in which the kidney was included in the irradiated area. This is, in general, a rare cause of kidney cancer.

GENETIC SUSCEPTIBILITY

There is some evidence that some cases of renal cell cancer may have a genetic basis. For example, there is increased risk of renal cancer in people with von-Hippel-Lindau's disease, a rare, dominantly inherited disorder. Further, there are several studies that suggest that several kidney tumour suppresser genes reside on the short arm of chromosome 3, although these genes are not a cause of familial heritability.

Suspected causes

CHEMICAL AGENTS

In some studies of coke production workers an increased risk of kidney cancer has been noted.

DIET

Several studies have shown that people with a high body mass index in the obese range have an increased risk for cancer of the body of the kidney. It is not clear if specific dietary factors are responsible for this increased risk. However, there is some evidence that those who consume plenty of fresh fruits and vegetables have a lower risk for kidney cancer. The cause of Wilm's tumours is not known.

Prevention

PRIMARY

The most important preventive action for kidney cancer is reduction of tobacco smoking. Abuse of analgesics should be avoided, especially those containing phenacetin. Promotion of ideal body weight will also reduce the risk of kidney cancer.

SECONDARY (EARLY DETECTION)

No screening test for kidney cancer is currently available.

Overall summary

Tobacco smoking causes approximately 40% of cancers of the body of the kidney and at least 60% of cancers of the renal pelvis. The proportion of cancers of the renal pelvis caused by phenacetin-containing analgesics in most countries is low (no more than 5%).

Chapter 15

Oral Cavity/Head and Neck Cancer

Cancers of the mouth or oral cavity and other parts of the head and neck are usually considered together because of their close proximity, the similarity of their causative agents, and the fact that the same group of clinical specialists, especially surgical and radiation oncologists, are involved in their treatment. For our purposes, the following sites will be considered together: lip, tongue, salivary glands, mouth, oropharynx, and hypopharynx.

An additional site, the nasopharynx, is often considered within the grouping of head and neck cancers, but because of major differences in its distribution in the world and in its causes, I consider it as a separate site in a subsequent chapter in this book.

Of this grouping of head and neck tumours, cancers of the lip and of the salivary glands show most differences from the rest, both in terms of their incidence internationally and because of differing causal factors. However, rather than describing them in separate chapters, I shall identify the relevant differences in the sections that follow.

There are, of course different parts of the mouth, including the gums, the floor of mouth under the front of the tongue, the hard and soft palates, and tonsils. These subsites are often coded separately in cancer registry data, although cancers arising in one section often spread to others, so precise classification is difficult. Beyond the palatal arch, the air we breathe and the food we eat pass into the pharynx. The oropharynx is encountered first, and then the hypopharynx. (The nasopharynx is above the oropharynx at the back of the nose.) Again, at times, precise localisation of cancers to these subsites may be difficult, and therefore there is another category (pharynx unspecified) combined into this grouping.

This grouping excludes a number of separate sites that are normally considered as falling within the head or neck. These include: the nose, nasal sinuses, and nasal passages; nasopharynx (as already mentioned); skull and brain; upper (cervical) spinal cord and the bones of the neck; the larynx; and the upper part of esophagus. The cancers arising in each of these parts of the head and neck are considered in separate chapters of this book.

Apart from cancers of the salivary glands and tonsils, the cancers that affect this grouping of sites are almost invariably squamous-celled. This is a reflection of the type of stratified epithelium lining the oral cavity and pharynx, which in practical terms is an extension of the skin.

Salivary gland tumours are different as they reflect the structure of these glands, which are responsible for the secretion of saliva into the mouth. Cancers that affect the tonsils also reflect the immune function of that organ and are usually cancers of lymphoid tissue and thus are usually considered with the lymphomas and separately classified. For this reason, we will not consider such cancers in this chapter.

The relative frequency of the main sites in the oral cavity and pharynx in males in Canada are: 17% lip, 20% tongue, 9% salivary gland, 18% mouth, and 36% pharynx, and 10%, 24%, 15%, 24%, and 27%, respectively, in females.

The head and neck cancers considered in this chapter are rare before the age of 40, and occur most frequently at ages of 50 or more.

Although incidence is lower in females than males, the relationship of increasing risk with increasing age is similar in both sexes.

There is a large variation in incidence reported from various registries—there are high rates in males in France and in both sexes in India; intermediate rates are reported in the US (but higher in US blacks than whites), Canada, and UK, and relatively low rates in Finland, Japan, and China. These differences reflect the prevalence of exposure to the major risk factors (see below). In general, there are similar variations between countries in death rates as for incidence, although the death rates are much lower than the incidence rates.

In general, the incidence of this grouping of cancers is relatively stable. The important exception is India, where the incidence of mouth cancer in both males and females has been falling. Mouth cancer incidence has also fallen in males in Finland, and recently in Canada and the US.

In Canada, the US, and the UK mortality from this group of cancers has been falling. In Denmark, however, there was quite a substantial rise in mortality, especially in males, and there was also a rise in Japan.

There is a range of survival internationally from more than 70% in North America in both males and females to less than 30% in females in Africa and Asia. Survival is best in oral cavity cancer, and poorest in cancer of the hypopharynx and survival is generally better in females than in males.

The natural history of these cancers has been studied largely with respect to cancer of the oral cavity, as the mucosa of the mouth is accessible to direct inspection and removal of cells from the lining of the mouth for microscopic examination. Precancerous changes in oral mucosa can often be detected by inspection. A white patch, or leukoplakia, is the appearance sought. The appearance may be apparently homogeneous or non-homogeneous. Leukoplakia is diagnosed when there is a white lesion of the oral mucosa with no apparent local cause such as friction, dental restoration, or cheek biting. The surface may be flat, corrugated, cracked or wrinkled; when non-homogeneous it may become indurated, nodular, erythematous (red-looking), or ulcerated.

The non-homogeneous changes are believed to be more advanced and are usually associated with epithelial dysplasia, a recognized precancerous change. They may become associated with changes throughout the thickness of the epithelium—carcinoma in situ. Carcinoma in situ may then be followed by the development of invasive carcinoma.

Exfoliated cells may show dysplastic changes and often the presence of micronuclei believed to be nuclear fragments that mark the later stages of oral carcinogenesis. Micronuclei are one of a group of precancerous biomarkers that can be used to monitor the effect of preventive approaches to cancer induction.

Proven causes of mouth and pharynx cancer

CHEMICAL AGENTS

The principal causes of mouth and pharynx cancer are tobacco and alcohol. Both smoking and chewing tobacco cause mouth cancer. Smoking tobacco causes cancer of the pharynx. Risk of both cancers increases with increasing intensity of cigarette smoking; per amount smoked the risk of pharynx cancer is higher than risk of mouth cancer. The risk associated with cigar or pipe smoking is lower than for cigarette smoking, but still greater than the risks incurred by non-smokers.

Similar dose/response relationships are seen for these sites with alcohol consumption. The level of alcohol consumption is much higher in France than the US, and the degree of risk associated with such consumption is correspondingly much greater. This helps to explain the much higher mortality from such cancers in France compared to other countries. Risk increases with all types of alcohol, but perhaps particularly from spirit consumption.

When the effects of both alcohol and tobacco are considered together it is found that they interact, and effectively one multiplies the effect of the other so that the risks of oral cavity and pharynx cancer become extremely high for heavy users of both tobacco and alcohol. There is increased risk with increasing consumption of alcohol and increasing smoking in non-smokers and non-drinkers, respectively. But the greatest risks, in the order of nearly a 16-fold increase, are seen in heavy drinkers and heavy smokers.

There is evidence that lip cancer risk is higher in heavy smokers, perhaps particularly smokers of pipes (and in the past, clay pipes) and heavy drinkers. The risk of salivary gland cancers, however, is unaffected by these exposures.

The chewing of tobacco, in a mixture with other substances, especially in India with betel nut and lime, has been associated with mouth cancer, which tends to develop in the area where the quid is placed, and is usually preceded by leukoplakia. Mixtures that include betel, but not tobacco also increase mouth cancer risk. Chewing tobacco appears to be increasing the risk of mouth cancer in North American native populations, particularly the Inuit of Canada, and also in Asian parts of the Russian Federation and neighbouring states. There is concern that tobacco preparations intended to be placed in the mouth ("snus", for example) will also increase the risk of mouth cancer.

Other uses of smoking also increase cancer risk. Thus the habit of reverse smoking in some parts of India, especially in women, where the lighted end of a type of cheroot or small cigar is placed inside the mouth, increases the risk of cancer of the hard palate.

PHYSICAL AGENTS

Sunlight exposure, especially in some occupations (fishing, agriculture, etc.) increases the risk of lip cancer.

Bad dentition is associated with increased risk of mouth cancer.

CHRONIC INFECTIONS

Infection with some subtypes of the human papilloma virus has been associated with increased risk of mouth cancer. There are many different subtypes of HPV. Those associated with mouth and perhaps pharynx cancer are the ano-genital types, the types also associated with cancer of the cervix. Possibly as much as 20% of mouth and pharynx cancers are due to infection with human papilloma viruses.

DIET AND NUTRITION

There is consistent evidence that the consumption of fruits and vegetables reduces the risk of mouth and pharynx cancers. In studies in Europe, North America, and Asia, it has been found that heavy consumers of vegetables and fruits have about half the risk of mouth and pharynx cancer as light consumers of these foods.

Suspected causes

DIET AND NUTRITION

Some studies have attempted to determine whether specific components of fruits and vegetables such as vitamin C and beta-carotene influence the risk of mouth and pharynx cancer. The evidence is slightly better for vitamin C, but in both instances it has been impossible to eliminate the possible protective effect of other substances in fruits and vegetables.

Studies in South America have suggested that the drinking of maté, a special tea drunk very hot through a straw, may increase the risk of oral cancer about twofold.

PHYSICAL AGENTS

There is increasing evidence that exposure to radiofrequency fields from use of mobile phones increases the risk of salivary gland cancers.

GENETIC SUSCEPTIBILITY

It seems probable that there is some genetic association with these cancers, but as yet, strong evidence has not emerged.

Prevention

PRIMARY

The most important preventive actions for mouth and pharynx cancers are reduction of alcohol consumption and cessation of cigarette smoking. In Asia, cessation of chewing of tobacco and/or betel mixtures is also important for protection against mouth cancer, while elsewhere it is important to recognize that chewing tobacco is not a safe alternative to cigarettes.

For lip cancer, protection against sunlight exposure is also very important.

There is no measure at present for protection against salivary gland cancers other than applying the precautionary principle in reducing use of mobile phones.

SECONDARY (EARLY DETECTION)

Screening for oral cancer by visual inspection has been advocated for high-risk areas such as India and other parts of Asia. There is evidence that subjects at high risk who already have the precancerous changes of leukoplakia can be identified. Visual inspection identifying high-risk subjects and urging them to stop smoking or chewing of tobacco and/or betel may also have an important role.

Overall summary

Tobacco use and alcohol consumption are the most important causes of cancer at these sites, accounting for the large majority of cases.

For lip cancer, however, sunlight causes about 50% of cases; alcohol and tobacco account for another 20% each.

For salivary gland cancer there are no known causes, but one suspected cause includes radiofrequency fields from mobile phones.

For mouth cancer, tobacco smoking and alcohol consumption, either separately or together, cause the majority of cases; chewing of tobacco in some areas (especially in Asia) are also major causes and poor dentition causes at least 10% of cases. Vegetable and fruit consumption reduces risk (low consumption increases risk and is responsible for about 20% of cases).

For pharynx cancer, smoking and alcohol and diet and nutrition have similar effects as for mouth cancer; chewing of tobacco and poor dentition are not causes.

Chapter 16

Nasopharynx Cancer

The nasopharynx is situated just behind the nose above the oropharynx. As explained in the previous chapter, this part of the pharynx is sufficiently different from the rest of the pharynx to justify separate consideration.

Nasopharyngeal carcinomas can vary from a highly differentiated squamous-celled carcinoma to an undifferentiated carcinoma that may resemble some types of malignant lymphoma. The latter can, however be distinguished by special stains. Adenocarcinomas may also occur. The characteristic nasopharyngeal carcinoma shows no evidence of mucin production or of glandular differentiation. It usually has a characteristic lymphoid stroma, and is sometimes called a lymphoepithelial carcinoma. The lymphocytes within its structure that may be numerous are in practice non-neoplastic (not malignant).

Nasopharyngeal carcinoma occurs in highest incidence in parts of China, or in migrant populations from China that were born in the high incidence areas of Southeast China adjacent to Hong Kong (the provinces of Guangdong, Guangxi, Hunan, and Fujian). Incidence is also high in Vietnam, some parts of North Africa, and among the Inuit populations of North America (Alaska and the

North West Territories of Canada) and Greenland. There are similar differences for mortality as for the incidence data.

The age distribution of cases of nasopharyngeal carcinoma shows a peak in incidence at about ages 50-60, and then a fall in both men and women. The fall with increasing age is more marked in high incidence Hong Kong than it is in Shanghai, or in the low incidence white population of the US. Incidence is higher in males than females in all areas.

In Hong Kong incidence is falling in both males and females, but in Singapore incidence is stable. In China and the Chinese populations living in Hawaii and the US, incidence is stable, or possibly falling. In developed countries the incidence rates are very low and stable.In Hong Kong there is 60% five-year survival in males and 66% in females. In Canada and other developed countries, survival is about 50% in both males and females.

Little is known of the natural history of these cancers. As yet, a detectable precursor lesion has not been identified.

Proven causes of nasopharyngeal cancers

CHEMICAL AGENTS

There is good evidence from a number of recent studies that tobacco smoking increases the risk of nasopharyngeal cancers. Although the elevation of risk for current smokers is less than for other cancers of the respiratory tract (in the order of a threefold increase in risk) this is similar to the risk for other non-respiratory cancers causally associated with tobacco smoking.

CHRONIC INFECTIONS

Chronic infection with the Epstein-Barr virus (EBV) is causally associated with the undifferentiated form of nasopharyngeal carcinoma. This virus is ubiquitous throughout the world. Infection is almost universal in some populations, infection being acquired in childhood. Although age at infection does not seem to be related to the risk of nasopharyngeal carcinoma, the virus can be found in virtually all cells of undifferentiated carcinomas and those with this form of the cancer have immunological evidence of infection with the virus.

DIET AND NUTRITION

Cantonese-style salted fish consumption is strongly associated with nasopharyngeal carcinoma. The highest risk has been found for consumption in infancy during weaning (in the order of eight- to 40-fold compared to non-consumers), with high risks also for consumption during childhood, but not in adult life. Cantonese-style salted fish is allowed to putrefy; it is its soft texture that makes it suitable for infant feeding. However, it has been demonstrated that this process results in the production of a carcinogen, one of the nitrosamines, and this seems to be the reason for the excess risk associated with the salted fish rather than with the salt itself.

Suspected Causes

CHEMICAL AGENTS

Occupational exposure to smoke and fumes has been associated with increased risk of nasopharyngeal cancer, especially in some studies in high-risk areas in Asia. Risk appears to be increased for exposure to dust and fumes and to non-tobacco smoke and also in one study from exposure to dusts, solvents and exhaust fumes. The elevation of risk in the exposed compared to the unexposed is in the order of two- to fourfold. Risk is also increased among woodworkers from exposure to wood dust.

Risk has also been associated with exposure to formaldehyde, which in the West can come from off-gassing from particle board, some plywoods, and forms of homes insulation no longer in use. Exposure from such sources was suspected as an explanation of the increased risk found in one study for people living in mobile homes.

DIET AND NUTRITION

There is some evidence from studies in high-risk populations that those with low consumption of fruits and vegetables are at increased risk of nasopharyngeal carcinoma.

Suspicion has also been placed on herbal tea consumption, but the evidence is very weak.

The diet of the Inuit used to include seal meat that was stored in the ground and allowed to putrefy. This meat appears to have been used for infant feeding. It is thus possible that this is the reason for the excess risk of nasopharyngeal carcinoma among Inuit populations, although no specific studies have been done as they have been for Chinese populations exposed to Cantonese-style salted fish.

There may also be a dietary cause for the increased risk of nasopharyngeal carcinoma in some African populations, but this has not yet been identified.

Prevention

PRIMARY

In Chinese populations at increased risk, the cessation of use of Cantonese-style salted fish, especially in infancy and childhood, is the most important preventive approach.

In Western populations, although risk is very low, tobacco control is likely to reduce risk.

Some benefit may also be derived by cleaning up work environments and ensuring adequate fruit and vegetable consumption.

SECONDARY (EARLY DETECTION)

There has been some interest in testing for high levels of antibodies to the Epstein-Barr virus in high-incidence Chinese populations. A difficulty is the ubiquity of such infection and the low specificity of the test. Such screening has not been shown to influence mortality from the disease.

Overall Summary

In high-incidence Chinese populations exposure to Cantonese-style salted fish appears to account for about 80% of the cases. Tobacco smoking may account for another 10% or so. Dietary factors are also probably important in other high-incidence populations.

In low-incidence populations only tobacco smoking is an established cause and is probably responsible for at least half of the cases that occur.

Chapter 17

Larynx Cancer

The larynx, or voice box, is situated in the neck, just beyond the lower part of the pharynx and just above the breathing tube or trachea. The larynx is sometimes considered in two parts, the upper or extrinsic larynx, and the lower or intrinsic larynx containing the vocal cords, with about two-thirds of the cancers involving the intrinsic larynx and usually the vocal cords. However, this distinction is not often made in terms of the causes of cancer of the larynx, nor is it maintained in routine data, so it will not be used here. The larynx is separated from the pharynx by a flap, the epiglottis, which prevents foods or liquids from entering the larynx when swallowing, but which moves up to allow air to enter and leave during breathing.

Almost all the cancers of the larynx are squamous-cell, reflecting the nature of the epithelium (stratified) lining the larynx, including the vocal cords.

The incidence of larynx cancer is much higher in men than women, and in the US is higher in blacks than whites. Although incidence rises with age, at older ages there is a downturn in incidence in most populations.

There is less variation in incidence and mortality from larynx cancer than for many other cancers, although rates are lower in Japan than the US, the UK, and Canada.

The trends in many countries almost certainly reflect the impact, varying with time, of the effects of alcohol and tobacco, the main causes of larynx cancer. (See below.)

In most countries, the five-year survival from larynx cancer approximates to 50%, although in some developing countries it is in the order of 20-20%, and in North America it is closer to 70%.

There is a carcinoma in situ phase of larynx cancer, although the disease is rarely detected in this stage, usually requiring the onset of symptoms, especially change of voice, for action to be taken that leads to its detection.

Proven causes of larynx cancer

CHEMICAL AGENTS

As implied earlier, tobacco smoking and heavy alcohol consumption are the dominant causes of cancer of the larynx. All forms of smoked tobacco increase risk; in most countries this usually implies cigarette smoking. But in some Asian countries other forms of tobacco are relevant, such as bidi smoking in India. In earlier studies it was felt that alcohol in the form of spirits especially increased risk; in more recent studies, all forms of alcohol have been implicated.

As for other cancers of the upper respiratory and gastro-intestinal tract (mouth, pharynx, esophagus), the effect of alcohol and tobacco together is to increase the risk substantially in a multiplicative (synergistic) interaction. For both non-smokers and non-drinkers the risk is very low. Those who are non-smokers but drink alcohol increase their risk of larynx cancer, the risk increasing with increasing consumption of alcohol. Similarly, for non-drinkers of alcohol who smoke, risk increases with increasing lifetime use of tobacco. The greatest risk, however, is incurred by those who are both heavy drinkers and heavy smokers.

Occupational exposures to strong inorganic acid mists containing sulphuric acid (such as in metal treatment, manufacture of batteries, and fertiliser production) increase the risk of larynx cancer in a dose-dependent manner. In a study in North America, mild exposure to such mists approximately doubled the risk of larynx cancer; heavy or intense exposure increased the risk more than sixfold.

The other occupational exposure now recognised as causally increasing the risk of larynx cancer is heavy and prolonged exposure to asbestos.

Suspected causes

CHEMICAL AGENTS

A number of chemicals or other agents encountered in the occupational environment have been suspected of causing larynx cancer, including nickel refining, coal tar pitches (in roofers and road workers), and isopropyl alcohol manufacture with the strong acid process. Of these, the evidence is least consistent for nickel exposure.

CHRONIC INFECTIONS

There is some evidence that the risk of larynx cancer may be increased by chronic infection with some types of the human papilloma virus.

DIET

High consumption of vegetables and fruits probably reduces the risk of larynx cancer. As yet, evidence for protective effects of specific foods and micronutrients is very weak.

Prevention

PRIMARY

The most important preventive actions are abolition of tobacco smoking, in whatever form exists in a country, and reduction in heavy alcohol consumption.

In industries where exposure has been shown to increase the risk of cancer of the larynx, efforts should be made to reduce exposure to the minimum.

SECONDARY (EARLY DETECTION)

No screening test is available for cancer of the larynx. Early detection will follow prompt recognition of the possibility of the cancer in those at risk, and appropriate diagnostic tests.

Overall summary

The proportion of larynx cancers explained by the two main risk factors—alcohol and tobacco—is over 80%, and in men closer to 90%. Occupational risk factors make a small contribution in the general population.

Chapter 18

Esophagus Cancer

The esophagus is the swallowing tube that runs from the back of the mouth through the chest to penetrate the diaphragm and terminate at the top end or "cardia" of the stomach. Cancers can occur at any position throughout the length of the esophagus and are generally described as occurring in the upper, middle, or lower third.

The majority of cancers occur in the epithelium or lining of the esophagus. Because the lining of the esophagus has to cope with undigested, sometimes hot food, the lining is usually similar to that described in other chapters of this book for external surfaces (especially the skin). Thus it is formed of squamous epithelium consisting of several layers of cells that grow to the surface and then slough off, or desquamate. Therefore, the majority of cancers that occur are squamous-celled carcinomas. However, in the lower part of the esophagus changes can occur in the epithelium to make it glandular-like, like the lining of the stomach. Then adenocarcinomas can occur.

Incidence is higher in males than females and increases progressively with age.

Esophageal cancer is the eighth most common cancer worldwide—with 455,780 new cases (3.2% of the total) estimated in

2012—and the sixth most common cause of death from cancer with 400,150 deaths (4.9% of the total). These figures encompass both adenocarcinoma and squamous-cell types. More than 80% of the cases and of the deaths occur in developing countries.

The incidence of esophageal cancer varies more than 15-fold in men and almost 20-fold in women internationally. Incidence is high in the Calvados region of France. However, the rates are probably higher in a belt of high esophageal cancer incidence that begins on the Southern shores of the Caspian sea and then stretches across Northern Iran, extending into the Southern Asian States of the former Soviet Union, then Eastward into Northern China. In Northern China it has been observed that there is also high incidence of esophageal cancer in chickens. It has been estimated that about half the cases of esophageal cancer in the world occur in China. In China, esophageal cancer is the second commonest cancer site, with stomach cancer number one. Esophageal cancer is also elevated in US blacks and in some South American countries, including parts of Brazil, Uruguay, and Argentina.

The highest mortality rates are found in both sexes in Eastern and Southern Africa and in Eastern Asia. There is a close similarity in the trends of incidence and mortality rates, showing increases in males and stability in females.

Survival from esophageal cancer is very low—no more than about 5% at five years in both males and females. This poor survival is very similar in Europe and most developing countries that have data.

The earliest changes that precede the development of squamous-cell cancer of the esophagus are dysplasia or atypical changes of the epithelium. This is followed by carcinoma in situ, then a fully invasive cancer. In subjects living in areas where there is a high risk for esophageal cancer, the earliest changes that can be detected by direct inspection of the esophageal mucosa are signs of inflammation, or esophagitis.

In the lower part of the esophagus changes in the epithelium sometimes occur associated with reflux of food from the stomach, especially when the muscle of the diaphragm is weakened. This can occur as a congenital or inherited effect or sometimes is acquired as a result of abdominal obesity. The resultant hernia through the diaphragm (or hiatus hernia, as it is called) allows food to regurgitate from the stomach into the esophagus and the epithelium of the lower esophagus undergoes changes so that it can cope with the partially digested, and now acid, food. The epithelium loses its squamous character, and becomes very similar to that of the stomach, a change that goes by the name Barrett's esophagus. This abnormal epithelium is susceptible to carcinogenic changes and adenocarcinomas (glandular type carcinomas) can then develop.

Proven causes of esophageal cancer

CHEMICAL AGENTS

In most developed countries, the predominant causes of squamous-cell esophageal cancer are tobacco smoking and alcohol drinking, similar to cancers of the head and neck. Risk is increased in alcohol drinkers who do not smoke, and in smokers who do not drink alcohol, but only to a small extent. The greatest increase in risk occurs in those who are both heavy drinkers and heavy smokers; indeed, the two risk factors interact in a multiplicative way, which is why they are considered together here.

Some of the areas with increased risk are clearly related to alcohol consumption, the most dramatic example being the increased risk in the Calvados region of France where local excess consumption of its namesake apple-based product results in the numbers of cases that occur.

Differences in racial or ethnic consumption patterns also result in risk differences, the much higher consumption of alcohol (including spirits) by US blacks being largely responsible for their higher risk than whites. In South Africa much of the increased risk in some areas is believed to be due to the high consumption of locally brewed alcoholic beverages, including kaffir beer.

Some of the changing trends in incidence and mortality described above may be due to changes in smoking and alcohol consumption. In general, alcohol consumption has not fallen to any great extent in the countries that have shown reductions in esophageal cancer; these reductions probably are largely due to changes in smoking. Many of the increases, however, may have been due to increase in alcohol consumption, an explanation believed probable in Denmark for their recent rises.

PHYSICAL AGENTS

In some parts of the world esophageal cancer is clearly related to the habit of drinking very hot (scalding) teas. For example, this has been demonstrated for Uruguay from the habit of drinking the beverage maté. Whether the effect is entirely due to the damage done by the scalding liquids to the lining of the esophagus is not clear, it is possible that some specific substances released by these hot teas may themselves be carcinogenic.

High occupational exposure to asbestos fibres increases risk about twofold, after a period of about 20 years.

The causes of the adenocarcinomas that occur in the lower part of the esophagus seem largely to be related to reflux of material from the stomach. Some of the cases are associated with congenital hiatus hernias that permit gastric reflux, although this is likely to be exacerbated by obesity.

DIET

A major cause of cancer at the lower end of the esophagus is excess caloric intake leading to obesity and gastric reflux.

There is convincing evidence that diets high in fruits and vegetables are protective for esophageal cancer. The evidence is strongest for green vegetables. Some studies also found protective effects for yellow vegetables and tomatoes. There is also evidence for protective effects when vegetables are eaten raw, as well as for citrus fruits. However, there is some evidence for increased risk of salt-pickled vegetables and limited or inconsistent evidence relating to root vegetables or tubers.

Genetic susceptibility

FAMILIAL CANCER SYNDROMES

Some families have been described in which there is an association between esophageal cancer and tylosis, a condition in which there is thickening of the palms and soles by keratosis. This seems to be rare and is not an explanation for the high rates in Asia.

Suspected causes

CHEMICAL AGENTS

In one high-risk area in Iran studies were performed many years ago in an attempt to identify the causes of the excess incidence of esophageal cancer. This was an area where poor nutrition was rife and it is also an opium smoking area. There was suspicion that the risk was increased from swallowing opium products (dross), products that have been shown to contain cancer-causing substances. However, because of the secrecy surrounding opium use, it was not possible to evaluate this hypothesis in detail. Nevertheless, some of the other high-risk areas of Asia are also areas where there is a tradition of opium use.

CHRONIC INFECTIONS

There is suspicion that infection with some oncogenic types of human papilloma viruses may increase the risk of esophageal cancer.

DIET

There is much indirect evidence that poor nutrition increases the risk of esophageal cancer. This may in part be responsible for the increased risk in high alcohol consumers in the West for example.

In most of the high-risk areas of the developing world the increased risk is clearly not associated with either alcohol or tobacco. Rather, cases occur in areas where there is much defective nutrition. It is not clear what nutritional deficiencies are responsible; some studies in high-risk areas of China have been performed when supplements containing some of the B vitamins were given to individuals living in those areas and the effect assessed on changes in the esophagus believed to precede the development of cancer. The studies did not succeed in reducing the prevalence of these changes. However, the occurrence of cancer was not assessed and it is possible that nutritional deficiencies have to be corrected earlier in life for an effect to occur.

In some parts of China increased risk appears to be associated with the consumption of mouldy corn or wheat due to contamination with a fungus.

GENETIC SUSCEPTIBILITY

It is possible that there are some forms of multigenic susceptibility that accounts for some of the differences in risk between different groups. However, the rates of esophageal cancer in Chinese that have migrated to Hawaii or Los Angeles are not especially high in comparison with non-migrants, so it seems probable that most of the international differences described above are due to environmental rather than genetic factors.

Prevention

PRIMARY

In Western populations, the most important preventive action for esophageal cancer is reduction in smoking and alcohol use, especially in combination. This, combined with increase in intake of vegetables and fruits and reduction in obesity would have a major impact on the risk of the disease.

In developing countries with areas of high risk it is likely, but not proved, that improvement in overall nutritional status would be of greatest benefit. In those areas, such as South Africa, where alcohol consumption is clearly related to increased risk, reduction in alcohol use can also be recommended. In addition, in countries where the habit is common drinking scalding teas should be actively discouraged.

SECONDARY (EARLY DETECTION)

There is no established screening method for esophageal cancer.

Overall summary

Ninety percent of squamous-cell esophageal cancers in the West can be explained by alcohol and tobacco consumption. The proportion also induced by low consumption of fruits and vegetables is probably in the order of 20-30% but clearly overlaps the effects of alcohol and tobacco. The major preventable cause of adenocarcinomas of the lower esophagus is obesity.

In developing countries, there is less certainty about the amount of disease accounted for by the risk factors discussed. Nevertheless, with adequate nutrition and avoidance of alcohol and tobacco it is likely that most of the disease could be prevented.

Chapter 19

Stomach Cancer

The stomach is the first receptacle for food in which digestion commences. Situated just under the diaphragm on the left toward the centre of the abdomen, it receives the masticated food from the esophagus and discharges it into the beginning of the small intestine (the duodenum) through a muscular tube (the pylorus). The top end of the stomach above the entrance of the esophagus (the gastroesophageal junction) is called the cardia, the main part of the body of the stomach.

Stomach cancers are also called gastric cancers, but the word stomach cancer is used in this book.

The healthy stomach excretes hydrochloric acid, which helps to kill any bacteria that enter the stomach. The stomach lining also excretes an agent that commences the process of digestion and which works in the acid environment of the stomach—an enzyme called pepsin.

There are two different types of stomach cancer—the intestinal and the diffuse varieties. The intestinal type is so called because of its resemblance to the epithelium of the rest of the intestine and the cells composing it are relatively large. It usually begins as a localised lesion that extends in all directions. It tends to be commoner

in older people and in males. Most of the differences in incidence
in different parts of the world (commented upon below) are due to
differences in the incidence of the intestinal type and the decrease
in incidence that has occurred in most countries is due to reduction in incidence of the intestinal type. In contrast, the diffuse type,
which represents a diffusely infiltrating lesion extending outward in
the mucosa, seems to be fairly constant in incidence in both space
and time. This type of cancer consists of small cells with a proliferation of the underlying connective tissue. It tends to be commoner in
younger than in older people and is equally frequent in males and
females.Although stomach cancer can occur in young people, it is
predominantly a disease of the elderly. Incidence is higher in males
than females, and in Japan compared to Canada, the US, the UK,
and other Western countries.

As recently as 1980 stomach cancer was estimated to be the most
common cancer in the world, accounting for about 650,000 cases
worldwide per year, or about 10.5% of all cancers. This number one
position had probably been held by stomach cancer for decades,
if not longer. The most recent estimate is for 2012, when almost
one million new cases of stomach cancer were estimated to have
occurred (951,600 cases, 6.8% of the total of all cancers), making it
the fourth most common malignancy in the world, behind cancers
of the lung, breast, and colorectum. More than 80% of cases (777,000
cases) occur in developing countries with almost twice as many in
men as in women, and half the world total occurs in Eastern Asia
(mainly in China). Incidence rates are about twice as high in men as
in women.

Stomach cancer is the second leading cause of cancer death in
both sexes worldwide (723,020 deaths in 2012, 8.8% of the total).
The highest mortality rates are estimated in Eastern Asia, the lowest
in North America. High mortality rates also occur in both sexes in
Central and Eastern Europe and in Central and South America.

The incidence of stomach cancer has been uniformly falling since
international records commenced in 1960; the registry with the

highest rates remains Japan (Miyagi) in both sexes, with a greater relative reduction in females. The lowest rates throughout were reported from India (Mumbai); this is a registry where the rates of esophageal cancer are higher than for stomach cancer.

The trends in mortality mirror those of incidence. However, over a longer time period, for some, but not all countries, the downward trend in mortality was delayed. Mortality was rising in the 1950s in Japan, Spain, and Portugal, Portugal being the last country to show a fall in mortality, and even now it has the highest rates in Western Europe. The country that showed the greatest decline was Finland; the rates for males and females were highest at the beginning of the period considered. In all countries the trends in females mirror those in males almost exactly, but the rates are lower. The lowest rates throughout in both males and females were seen in the US.

For some countries, Canada, the UK, and the US, for example, data are available on mortality from stomach cancer in the 1930s. At that time stomach cancer was uniformly the most important cause of cancer death in those countries, holding the position that lung cancer came to hold in the 1980s.

Survival relative to that of people of the same age and sex is low for stomach cancer, both in Europe and North America, being just under 20% at five years for males, and just over 20% for females. In Canada, the five-year relative survival increased from 19% in 1992-94 to 25% in 2005-07. In developing countries the best reported survival was from Shanghai—slightly better than developed countries, but elsewhere five-year relative survival approximated to 10%, sometimes with higher survival in males than females.

The process of carcinogenesis in the stomach probably begins with the development of chronic inflammation of the stomach lining, or chronic gastritis. In high-risk areas chronic gastritis occurs even in children. This is eventually accompanied by an inability of the cells in the stomach to produce hydrochloric acid (an achlorhydric state), so that the stomach becomes even more susceptible to inflammation. With rapid turnover of cells caused by this inflammatory process, the opportunity for error in cell division increases, with the possibility that one cell will be so changed that it begins a process of abnormal cell division, with cells replicated in its own image. A succession of such clonal changes is probably required for stomach cancer to eventually develop. These steps in the development of stomach cancer have not been as well identified as they have for colon cancer.

Proven causes of stomach cancer

CHEMICAL AGENTS

Smoking is associated with an increased risk of stomach cancer; the increase seen is relatively modest.

PHYSICAL AGENTS

In several studies, intense occupational exposure to asbestos fibres has been found to increase the risk of stomach cancer about twofold, after a lag period of about 20 years. This is almost certainly causal, although the number of cases induced by asbestos in the population as a whole is probably very few.

High levels of radiation increased the risk of stomach cancer in the victims of the atomic bomb explosions in Japan, and also in some medically exposed populations that had high levels of radiation to the abdomen.

CHRONIC INFECTIONS

The organism *Helicobacter pylori* is a spiral flagellated gram-negative bacterium that can colonize human gastric mucosa and survive in the acid environment of the stomach. *H. pylori* infection is the main cause of chronic gastritis, and also of peptic ulcer. Serological evidence of infection with *H. pylori* has been associated in several studies with increased risk of stomach cancer, and is considered to be a cause of stomach cancer. However, it is probably not a necessary or sufficient cause of stomach cancer, as stomach cancer can occur in the absence of evidence of *H. pylori* infection, and only a small proportion of those infected eventually develop stomach cancer.

DIET

There is strong and consistent evidence that diets low in fruit and vegetable consumption, especially of non-starchy vegetables, increase the risk of stomach cancer, as does the absence of refrigeration. The protective effect of refrigeration probably relates to facilitation of the year-round availability of fruits and vegetables, and reducing the need for salt and nitrite used in food preparation. Citrus fruits are strongly linked to protective effects, while raw vegetables and vegetables of the allium type (onion and garlic, for example) are also protective. Salted and pickled vegetables, however, are not protective.

Several specific dietary factors are associated with the risk of stomach cancer. These include consumption of nitrites and salt in preserved foods increasing risk, and a protective effect of vitamin C. Salt probably increases risk by inducing or aggravating chronic gastritis while nitrite can interact with products of protein in the stomach (amines) producing carcinogenic nitrosamines, a reaction that is inhibited by vitamin C. Nitrate can be broken down to nitrite in the saliva. When nitrate is taken into the body as constituents of certain vegetables, the presence of vitamin C in the vegetable prevents the induction of stomach cancer. However, when nitrate consumption is unaccompanied with vitamin C, as in excess nitrate in drinking water, it can increase the risk of stomach cancer.

GENETIC SUSCEPTIBILITY

Cancer of the stomach occurs slightly more often among persons with blood type A than among those with other types. It is also increased in those who suffer from a hereditary form of atrophic gastritis.

Suspected causes

CHRONIC INFECTIONS

Infection with the Epstein-Barr virus (EBV) is suspected of being a cause of up to one-third of stomach cancers, especially those with, but not restricted to, lymphocyte infiltration. EBV tends to be ubiquitous, so there must be other factors that lead to its incorporation in the cells of the gastric mucosa and stimulation of the carcinogenic process; these have not yet been identified.

DIET

Dietary factors that may increase the risk of stomach cancer include high starch consumption and grilled or barbecued meat. Factors that may be protective include whole grain cereals and green tea consumption. No relationship has been found with black tea consumption and alcohol use.

PREVIOUS MEDICAL HISTORY

There has been a suspicion that a history of gastric ulcer is associated with increased risk of stomach cancer. The evidence has been inconsistent, except for those treated by surgery involving an anastomosis of the stomach with the small intestine, as occurs when the pylorus is resected or by-passed (gastro-enterostomy). Gastric ulcers are associated with and probably caused by *H. pylori* infection. Thus the mechanism of risk following surgery for gastric ulcer may be an exacerbation of chronic gastritis.

Genetic susceptibility

FAMILIAL CANCER SYNDROMES

No specific familial syndromes for stomach cancer have been identified. Those with a family history of stomach cancer are at increased risk compared to those without such a history. However, it is possible that this is due to shared exposure to environmental factors rather than an inherited predisposition to stomach cancer.

Prevention

PRIMARY

The most important preventive action for stomach cancer appears to be promotion of high fruit and vegetable consumption. Although this cannot now be proved, it seems very likely that the availability of refrigeration, and thus the increased availability of fruits and vegetables, has been largely responsible for the major declines in stomach cancer that have occurred.

H. pylori infection can be eradicated by antibiotic use. The extent to which the decline of stomach cancer can be attributed to the widespread use of antibiotics for other infections cannot be determined, but it may have contributed. At present, there is no policy for deliberate eradication of *H. pylori* infection by using antibiotics, except in some subjects judged clinically to be at high risk. The effect of such a program has not been evaluated.

SECONDARY (EARLY DETECTION)

Screening for stomach cancer using standardized photofluorographic (X-ray) examinations of the stomach is policy in Japan. It is still not clear whether this has contributed to the decline in mortality from stomach cancer in Japan. However, some recent studies have suggested a minimal effect while a special study of the Japanese approach to screening in a high-risk area of Venezuela found no benefit. Therefore, screening for stomach cancer is not recommended in countries outside Japan.

Overall summary

The proportion of stomach cancers explained by the various risk factors discussed above, especially lack of fruit and vegetable intake, absence of refrigeration, low intake of vitamin C and high intake of nitrite and salt, is probably as high as 80%. The additional (overlapping) risk contributed by *H. pylori* infection is unknown, but may be as high as 60%.

Chapter 20

Liver Cancer

The liver, situated in the upper abdomen under the diaphragm and lower rib cage on the right, is an essential organ for the metabolism of ingested substances from foods, and for the detoxification of potentially harmful substances. Life is not possible without a functioning liver. It is a very vascular organ and its blood supply comes directly from both the heart via the hepatic artery and from the intestine via the portal vein. After the liver cells have done their work the products are excreted back into the circulation through the hepatic vein. This efficient system means that toxic products absorbed from the intestine do not get into the general circulation— they are detoxified first in the liver. The liver is also a reservoir of glycogen, the storage medium of sugars; if blood glucose level falls the liver puts more glucose into the circulation.

The liver excretes the products of its metabolism into the intestine through the bile duct system for discharge in the feces. Bile does not only act as a medium of excretion, it also contains bile salts produced by the liver that facilitate digestion, especially of fats. If the bile duct system is obstructed so that bile cannot reach the intestine, the bile refluxes into the hepatic venous system, and the person becomes jaundiced (yellow). Jaundice can also occur when the bile duct system is temporarily damaged by inflammation, as in infection with the hepatitis A virus.

Unfortunately, the liver, although capable of regeneration, can be permanently damaged both by certain types of viruses (especially the hepatitis B and C viruses) and by certain toxins, especially chronic alcohol ingestion. This damage is usually expressed initially by inflammation (hepatitis), and then if damage continues, by the replacement of liver tissue by fibrous tissue, a condition called cirrhosis of the liver. There is considerable reserve capacity in the normal liver. However, the reserve capacity in the cirrhotic liver is low, and if it is exceeded liver failure, jaundice, and death will supervene.

Two types of cancers can occur primarily in the liver. The most common is primary hepatocellular carcinoma arising in the liver cells themselves. It is this type of liver cancer to which we mainly refer to as liver cancer.

The other type of primary liver cancer arises in the cells of the bile duct system and is called cholangiocarcinoma. Less is known of this type of liver cancer, although in one area of the world where cholangiocarcinomas are more frequent, there is a specific cause. In the sections below, I shall only refer to cholangiocarcinomas when I can refer to a specific cause. The causes of those rare cholangiocarcinomas that occur in most countries are unknown.

Occasionally, sarcomas, or blood vessel cancers (haemangiosarcomas) occur in the liver. With the exception of one specific cause for haemangiosarcoma, the causes of these cancers are unknown.

Primary liver cancers have to be distinguished from cancers that have metastasized (spread through the bloodstream) from primary sites elsewhere, especially the intestines and organs in the abdomen, breast, and lung, although all cancers that metastasize (except those of the brain) can spread to the liver. Many people who are said to have died of liver cancer have in fact not had a primary liver cancer but a secondary spread from another site. It can sometimes be difficult, unless detailed investigations are done, to distinguish clinically between a secondary liver cancer and a primary liver cancer. In general, this is now done with some accuracy in developed countries, but may have not been so accurate in the past; therefore, trend data have to be interpreted circumspectly. In the developing countries where primary liver cancer is common, however, the other cancers that can metastasize to the liver are less common and we can have confidence in the differences that are reported.

The incidence of liver cancer increases steadily with increasing age, both in countries with high rates of liver cancer (for example, China) and in countries with low rates such as Canada and the US. The disease occurs in children, but the rates are very low. Rates are higher in males than females, but still much higher in females in high incidence areas than in low.In 2012 liver cancer was the fifth most common cancer in men in the world (554,370 cases, 7.5% of the total) and the seventh in women (228,000 cases, 3.1% of the total). Most of the burden was in developing countries where almost 85% of the cases occur, particularly in men. The regions of high incidence are Eastern and Southeastern Asia, Middle and Western Africa, and also Melanesia and Micronesia/Polynesia, particularly in men. Low rates are estimated in developed regions, with the exception of Southern Europe where the incidence in men is significantly higher than in other developed regions.

There were an estimated 745,500 deaths from liver cancer in the world in 2012 (over twice as many in men as in women) and because of its high fatality (overall ratio of mortality to incidence of 0.93), liver cancer is the third most common cause of death from cancer worldwide. In a special study of survival from liver cancer in some developing countries where liver cancer was relatively common, it was found that the majority of deaths occurred within six months and that very few patients with liver cancer were alive after 12 months. In Canada, there has been an improvement in survival from liver cancer, from a five-year survival of 10% in 1992-94 relative to the survival of people free of liver cancer of similar age and sex to one of 18% in 2005-07.

The early stage of cancer development in the liver appears to be the occurrence of foci of altered liver cells (hepatocytes) preceding the development of both benign and malignant liver tumours. Benign liver tumours, or hepatomas, may develop from these altered liver cells, but it is not certain that adenomas always precede the development of malignant tumours, the primary hepatocellular carcinomas, which seem to be able to arise de novo from the altered hepatocytes.

There is a strong association between the occurrence of inflammatory fibrous changes in the liver (cirrhosis) and the development of primary hepatocellular carcinomas.

Proven causes of liver cancer

CHEMICAL AGENTS

Alcohol is an important cause of liver cancer, especially in developed countries. In practice, it is chronic alcohol abuse over many years that leads to increased risk of liver cancer, with the intermediate development of liver fibrosis or cirrhosis. As cirrhosis can itself lead to liver failure and death, alcoholics who develop liver cancer almost always have major impairments of liver function, which complicates therapy and often contributes to death.

An occupational cause for a rare form of liver cancer is exposure to vinyl chloride during the production of some forms of plastics. This was first identified by the occurrence of a cluster of haemangiosarcomas of the liver in a plastic manufacturing plant in the US; cases were subsequently found to have occurred in similar plants elsewhere. The occurrence of this cancer was prevented after new manufacturing processes were introduced that ensured that there was no exposure of workers to the raw vinyl chloride.

PHYSICAL AGENTS

Patients who were injected for diagnostic purposes with a radioactive isotope thorium-232 (Thorotrast) had a high frequency of cholangiosarcomas and haemangiosarcomas. Thorotrast is no longer used, but the survivors (largely in parts of continental Europe), continue to show high rates of these cancers.

CHRONIC INFECTIONS

Chronic infection with the hepatitis B virus (HBV) is an established major cause of primary hepatocellular carcinoma, especially in Asia and Africa. Those at high risk are chronic carriers of the virus, as identified by the presence in their blood of hepatitis B antigen. Liver cancer occurs years after infection has occurred, usually in association with cirrhosis consequent on the inflammation and fibrosis that are caused by the virus. Transmission of the virus appears to largely occur from mother to child in Asia, and from child to child at young ages in Africa. HBV can also be transmitted through infected blood and probably also by sexual intercourse. It has therefore become a major risk among drug addicts when they use needles that have been shared with others who are infected.In Japan, and also in other parts of the world including Canada and the US, an important cause of liver cancer is chronic infection with the hepatitis C virus (HCV). This virus, which used to be called nonA-nonB, is the agent that causes transfusion hepatitis; it is largely caused by the transfer of infected blood products to humans. Again, the mechanism for the production of cancer is the development of cirrhosis.

In parts of Southeast Asia, where liver cancer is relatively common, approximately 60% of such cancers are cancers of the bile ducts (Cholangiocarcinoma). The cause appears to be infestation with a parasite, the liver fluke (either *Clonorchis sinensis or Opisthorcis viverrini).* Cholangiocarcinomas are rare in developed countries, and those that occur are not due to parasites.

DIET

A number of studies correlating estimates of the incidence of primary liver cancer with the intake of aflatoxin (a naturally occurring mycotoxin produced by a fungus that can contaminate mouldy grain and other foods) in the same population groups have been performed. The incidence of liver cancer differs substantially between as well as within these areas; this variation in incidence is strongly correlated with differences in the estimated intake of aflatoxin.

Studies in Africa in which differences in liver tumour incidence by area were evaluated simultaneously with area data on aflatoxin exposure and hepatitis B infection have found that aflatoxin exposure appeared to be more important than hepatitis B infection in explaining the variation in liver cancer incidence. Similarly, in China a number of studies have been performed correlating liver cancer incidence or mortality with estimates of aflatoxin exposure by area, and several have attempted to take hepatitis B infection into account. In several studies differences in liver cancer rates did not seem to be explained by differences in hepatitis B infection, but were explained by differences in aflatoxin exposure. In one large study, the reverse was found. However, when it was possible to measure both factors accurately it seemed that aflatoxin-contaminated foods increased the risk in both individuals who did and did not have evidence of chronic hepatitis B infection; the greatest risk of liver cancer occurred in those with evidence of both exposures. As a result of such studies, aflatoxin is accepted as a human carcinogen.

A study of cholangiocarcinoma in Thailand did not find evidence of increased risk from aflatoxin exposure.

Suspected causes

CHEMICAL AGENTS

There is some evidence of an association of primary liver cancer with long-term use of oral contraceptives. Such cancers are rare, but may be preceded by the development of hepatomas, which have also been associated with use of oral contraceptives.

There is some evidence that occupational exposure to trichlorethylene (in dry cleaning) is associated with an increased risk of liver cancer.

DIET

A protective effect of high fruit and vegetable intake for liver cancer has been found in studies in Italy.

Prevention

PRIMARY

In the West, the most important preventive action for liver cancer is avoiding chronic alcoholism and the development of cirrhosis. Steps have largely been taken to avoid transmission of HCV through blood products, but HBV transmission in drug addicts continues, requiring needle exchange programs to diminish transmission, as for the human immunodeficiency virus (HIV).In Asia and Africa inclusion of vaccination against the hepatitis B virus in the expanded program of immunization in children would be the most important action to take. Such programs have become routine in the wealthy countries of these regions, but have hardly been initiated in many areas where the need is greatest. It is estimated that fewer than 10% of those at risk of liver cancer have yet been vaccinated. The difficulty is that for a major impact it will be necessary to wait at least 30 years before a protective effect upon liver cancer is seen, and the maximum impact will not occur for 50 years. However, liver cancer prevention is not the only benefit from hepatitis B vaccination programs; reduction in childhood hepatitis and adult cirrhosis would also follow successful vaccination campaigns.

SECONDARY (EARLY DETECTION)

Screening for liver cancer has been attempted in some experimental programs in China and Japan. Although there was some increase in the proportion of cases in stage 1 and a reduction of those in stage 3, such changes could not be expected to have much impact on deaths from the disease. Thus, therapy for detected cancers is problematic given the late stage of many of the cancers detected, so screening cannot be recommended at the present time.

Overall summary

In the West, the proportion of liver cancers explained by the known risk factors (alcohol, HCV infection) approximates to 70%. In Asia and Africa probably over 80% of cases are caused by aflatoxin-contamination of food and/or chronic infection with the HBV. However, the relative contribution of these two causes varies from region to region. In Northeast Thailand about 60% of liver cancers are cholangiocarcinomas, caused by liver flukes.

Chapter 21

Gall Bladder and Bile Duct Cancers

The gall bladder is situated on the underside of the liver on the right side of the abdominal cavity. It is the receptacle for the storage of bile, which is an important contributor to the process of digestion of fats in the intestine. The liver excretes bile; it passes through the intrahepatic (within the liver) bile ducts to the gall bladder where it is stored and concentrated. When bile is required for digestion, the gall bladder contracts, and the bile passes down the common bile duct to enter the duodenum (upper part of the small intestine, just beyond the stomach) at the ampulla of Vater.

Cancers can develop in the gall bladder, the common bile duct, and the intrahepatic ducts. Those that develop in the intrahepatic ducts are called cholangiocarcinomas and are described in the chapter on liver cancer.

Gall bladder cancers are usually adenocarcinomas, representing the glandular structure of the epithelium (lining) of the gall bladder. Sometimes they may become papillary in appearance. Rarely, gall bladder cancers are epidermoid, or squamous-cell. Bile duct cancers are also adenocarcinomas.

In international data, these cancers, with the exception of the cancers of the intrahepatic bile ducts, are usually grouped together and will be so considered in the rest of this chapter. The majority of the cancers are of the gall bladder, however.

Gall bladder and bile duct cancers occur with approximately the same frequency in women and in men. It is largely a disease of old age. Incidence is higher in Japan than in Canada, the US, and UK. The disease also seems to occur more frequently in Italy than other parts of Europe. Survival is in the order of 60% at five years for both males and females in Canada, the UK, and US, although lower in Japan.

PROVEN CAUSES OF GALL BLADDER CANCER

The only proven and probably causal association for gall bladder cancer is the relationship to gallstones. The majority (60-70%) of subjects with gall bladder cancer have gallstones, which tend to be cholesterol stones in the West and pigment stones in Asian countries. In the US, 10% to 15% of adult males and 25% of females have gallstones.

Obesity is a risk factor for gallstones, and in their turn, for gall bladder cancer.

Suspected causes

DIET

The few studies that have been done suggest that high fat and possibly cholesterol intake may increase the risk of gall bladder cancer, and that intake of fruits and vegetables may be protective.

In one study, alcohol intake appeared to increase the risk of bile duct cancer, but not gall bladder cancer.

Prevention

Reduction in obesity is probably protective for gall bladder cancer.

Overall summary

Other than gallstones, the causes of gall bladder cancer are largely unknown. The proportion of gall bladder cancers explained by gallstones and obesity approximates to 60%.

Chapter 22

Pancreas Cancer

The pancreas is an organ that lies at the back of the abdomen, nestling in the curve of the duodenum into which the pancreatic duct empties. The pancreas consists of a head, a body, and a tail that reach across the back of the abdomen from right to left. The pancreas has as its main function the production of digestive juices (enzymes) that function in relation to the digestion and absorption of food as it passes from the duodenum, the first part of the small intestine beyond the stomach, into the jejunum and ilium, the next parts of the small intestine. The part of the pancreas that contributes to this function is sometimes called the exocrine pancreas (i.e., the part of the pancreas that excretes enzymes outside the pancreas into the duodenum). However, the pancreas also has within it what are called the islets of Langerhans. These produce the hormone insulin, secreted into the bloodstream to facilitate the deposition of glucose from the blood into the organs that require it for functioning, and these islets comprise the endocrine part of the pancreas. Tumours of the islets can occur—these are marked by an over-excretion of insulin and severe symptomatology, but are rare. They tend to have a better prognosis than the cancers of the exocrine pancreas.

Interference with the endocrine function of the pancreas results in diabetes.

The main cancers of the exocrine pancreas are glandular-like (adenocarcinomas). About two-thirds arise in the head of the pancreas, the remainder in the body and tail.

Pancreas cancer is mainly a disease of the elderly with incidence rates increasing progressively with age. Rates are higher in males than females, although the differences are not great.

Although rates are lower in Africa and Asia than in Europe and the Americas, the differences between Europe and the Americas are much less than for many other cancers. Rates of incidence and mortality are very similar. In males, generally with somewhat higher rates than females, the rates are highest in Eastern Europe and in females in North America.

In males in North America and Europe incidence has fallen after an initial rise. But for Japan (Miyagi) there has been an important rise. These trends probably reflect changes in the impact of the major risk factor, tobacco smoking (see below). For females the trends in incidence have almost universally shown an increase, again probably reflecting the impact of the tobacco epidemic. However, rates in India in both sexes are low. Trends in mortality have mirrored the trends in incidence.

Survival from pancreas cancer is very poor, with most cases dying within six months and nearly all within a year of diagnosis. These dismal figures represent the difficulties in diagnosis and the late (advanced) stage at which nearly all diagnoses are made.

The natural history of pancreas cancer is unknown, with no precursor lesion as yet recognised. However, many believe the cancers arise from the small ducts within the pancreas that collect digestive juices. There is a relationship with diabetes, which in many studies appears to be a risk factor, although the mechanism for such an effect is unclear.

Proven causes of pancreas cancer

CHEMICAL AGENTS

The most important established cause for pancreas cancer is tobacco smoking. The risk among smokers is two to three times the risk in non-smokers, with heavy cigarette smokers acquiring a sixfold increased risk. Ex-smokers have a lower risk, although, like lung cancer, the extent of the risk is dependent on how long they have smoked and it does not seem to return to normal.

PHYSICAL AGENTS

Ionising radiation, especially medical irradiation that directly involves the pancreas (for example, patients treated for ankylosing spondylitis) increases the risk of pancreas cancer.

OBESITY

Obesity (both body fatness and abdominal fatness) is associated with increased risk of pancreas cancer. Risk is also increased in those with greater adult-attained height.

Chronic inflammation

There is an association between a history of pancreatitis (an inflammatory condition of the pancreas) and pancreatic cancer. This should probably not be regarded as a chronic infection. It appears to be the idiopathic (cause unknown) pancreatitis that increases risk, not the form of pancreatitis associated with alcohol consumption.

Suspected causes

CHEMICAL AGENTS

Certain occupational exposures have been suspected of increasing the risk of pancreas cancer, especially chronic exposure to pesticides, but also to hydrocarbon solvents and metal working fluids.

DIET

A number of dietary factors have been found to be associated with pancreas cancer. High energy intake was found to increase risk in a dose-dependent manner in three studies, but not in every study. The main determinant of energy that increased risk was carbohydrate intake, especially of sugars. In other studies, dietary cholesterol has also been found to increase risk, as well as meat. High fruit and especially vegetable intake appear to reduce risk; specific micronutrients, including beta-carotene, have not yet been reliably implicated. However, foods containing folate appear to be protective.

GENETIC SUSCEPTIBILITY

There is some evidence of familial susceptibility, but familial cancer syndromes exclusively involving the pancreas are unknown.

Unproven causes

CHEMICAL AGENTS

In the past, suspicion has been raised that chronic alcohol intake—and in other studies, coffee drinking—is associated with risk of pancreas cancer. More recently, sufficient studies have been conducted finding no association with pancreas cancer to permit the conclusion that neither alcohol nor coffee intake increases the risk of pancreas cancer.

Prevention

PRIMARY

The most important primary prevention measure for pancreas cancer is reduction in tobacco smoking. As implied above, there is some evidence that reduction in smoking in some Western countries is already leading to a reduction in pancreas cancer, especially in males.

SECONDARY (EARLY DETECTION)

No screening test for pancreas cancer is available.

Overall summary

In countries that have experienced the full force of the tobacco epidemic the proportion of pancreas cancers explained by smoking is in the order of 40% or more in males and 25% in females. However, in view of the dramatic changes in incidence and mortality that have occurred, explicable only by the progress of the tobacco epidemic, these figures may be underestimates, with possibly at least 50-60% in males and 40% in females explicable due to smoking.

If dietary factors are causal (at present these are not yet established as causes), it is likely that diet explains at least another 40% of pancreas cancer.

Chapter 23

Malignant Melanoma of the Skin

Malignant melanoma of the skin is the most fatal form of skin cancer. (The other forms are described in the following chapter.) Malignant melanomas also occur in the eye, but as these are usually classified with other tumours of the eye they will be discussed in the chapter on cancers of the eye. Malignant melanomas of the skin can occur on any part of the skin surface. For simplicity, in the remainder of this chapter melanoma will be used to refer to malignant melanoma of the skin.

Four types of melanoma have been described. Superficial spreading melanoma and nodular melanoma tend to occur in younger people, and are commonest in fair-skinned populations. Superficial spreading melanoma accounts for more than 50% of melanomas. Nodular melanomas are the next most common; they may derive from areas of superficial spreading melanoma that have gone undetected. Lentigo melanoma tends to occur in older people with sun-damaged skin. This is rare, and most commonly occurs on the head and neck. Acral lentiginous melanoma tends to occur on the soles of the feet and sometimes the palms and appears to be a reaction to trauma, occurring rarely in Caucasians, but more frequently, though rarely, in Africans.

Melanomas are derived from the melanin-producing cells (melanocytes) situated in the deeper layers of the skin. Melanin (pigment) protects tissues below the skin from the harmful effects of ultraviolet light exposure. Melanocytes tend to become active or multiply with sun exposure in fair-skinned populations. With exposure to ultraviolet light there may be an immediate skin darkening due to release of melanin from melanocytes. With delayed tanning there is an increase in the number of melanocytes as well as an increase in their activity. Dark-skinned populations have many more melanin-producing cells that cover extensive areas of the deeper layers of the skin than fair-skinned populations; these are responsible for the natural protection to sunlight that these populations possess. In fair-skinned populations, freckles and larger pigment-containing areas in the skin, or nevi, appear in response to exposure to sunlight. In some of these nevi, dysplastic changes (multiplication and cell change) occur and these are believed to be the first stages in the development of melanomas. Immunological factors appear to have some influence on the development of dysplastic nevi. In some individuals, immunological activity may produce a halo effect of loss of pigment around the nevus, often presaging the disappearance of the early possibly dysplastic nevus. Such individuals appear to have a built-in protective effect against the development of melanoma.

The risk of melanoma increases with advancing age. In the US rates are much higher in whites than blacks. There is a large variation in incidence worldwide, for both males and females. The highest incidence by a substantial margin is in Australasia, driven by high rates in Australia, and to a lesser extent in New Zealand, the lowest in most developing countries and in Asia. High rates, but still much lower than in Australasia, are also seen in North America and Europe, with the highest in Europe in Northern Europe. Mortality mirrors these differences, but in all areas incidence is substantially greater than mortality.

Fair-skinned populations that have migrated from an area of relatively low sun exposure to one of high (such as migrants from the UK to Australia) show a much higher incidence of melanoma than those in the originating country. In general, risk increases with the duration of residence in the host country. Those who migrate as children, or who are born of immigrant parents in the host country of their parents, tend to show an even higher risk.

The incidence of melanoma has increased dramatically in Australia and to a lesser extent in North America and many European populations. Mortality has not increased to the same extent as incidence; this has led to the suspicion that some of the increase in incidence is caused by a greater awareness of the risk in fair-skinned populations, and that therefore part of the increase is due to early detection, and even over-diagnosis, of some lesions. Nevertheless, in males, mortality has been rising consistently. For females, however, in relatively low mortality countries such as Canada, mortality has stabilised in recent years and may be beginning to fall. In Australia, mortality is much higher in males than females; in other countries it is very similar.

Survival from melanoma is relatively good, especially for those cases with limited extent of invasion into the dermis of the skin, just below the epidermis. However, survival is much inferior to other forms of skin cancer where mortality from the disease is rare. Survival is better for cases of superficial spreading melanoma than for nodular melanoma. In the US, five-year survival, relative to that for the general population, is 85% for white males and 91% for white females. In Canada the relative five-year survival for males and females combined increased a little from 84% in 1992-94 to 89% in 2005-07.

Proven causes of malignant melanoma

PHYSICAL AGENTS

Exposure to sunlight (ultraviolet light) is the principal cause of melanoma. However, the nature of the exposure and its relationship to constitutional (innate) factors was not originally understood. Indeed, the common sites for melanoma, such as the trunk, are not normally exposed to sunlight, except with recreational pursuits. This is what gave the clue to causation. Those at greatest risk of melanoma are those constitutionally liable to sunburn, especially if they have had episodes of severe sunburn in childhood or adolescence. Further, it is the sites on the skin where sunburn tends to occur where the risk is greatest.

Those with occupational exposure to sunlight, such as road and construction workers, have if anything a lower risk of melanoma, quite different from their increased risk for other forms of skin cancer. This is probably in part a self-selection phenomenon; those people with light skin, constitutionally at greater risk of melanoma, would not be likely to enter an occupation where they were liable to develop severe and painful sunburn. So it is those with dark skin that tend to self-select for such occupations, largely explaining their lower risk of melanoma.

GENETIC SUSCEPTIBILITY

As indicated above, constitutional risk associated with intermittent or recreational sun exposure is the principal cause of melanoma. Constitutional risk, apart from the susceptibility to sunburn, occurs largely in those populations who originally chose to live in northern regions, especially Nordic peoples and those descended from the Angles. This constitutional risk is exhibited by fair skin, light hair, blue eyes, and inability to tan following sun exposure. The people in those areas of the world to which such people have migrated, including North America, Australia, and New Zealand also show constitutional risk. There is no question that such susceptibility is inherited, although the genes responsible have not been identified. The risk is expressed especially when exposure to sunlight occurs in childhood. Thus, those with constitutional predisposition who experienced excess sun exposure as new migrants as adults have half the risk of those with the same constitutional background who migrate as children or those who are born in the country to which their forebears migrated.

In those constitutionally predisposed to increased risk of melanoma, an index of sun exposure that correlates well with acquired melanoma risk is the number of acquired melanocytic nevi on the forearms.

Those who have historically resided in areas of greater sunlight than in northern latitudes tend to have inherited features that protect them against melanoma: dark skin, dark hair, brown eyes, and ability to tan readily on exposure. These are principally those who live around the Mediterranean basin in Europe, in India, Africa, and Asia. In addition, those peoples who have descended from the Celts in the UK seem to have lower risk. Of course, with time much genetic admixture has occurred among such peoples, but it is usually obvious which are at greatest risk, and which least.

FAMILIAL CANCER SYNDROMES

There is some indication of familial susceptibility to melanoma. This is principally, but not entirely, manifested by those with the dysplastic nevi syndrome. The dysplastic nevi syndrome represents a familial tendency to develop atypical pigmented nevi on the skin, which on biopsy are already found to show cellular changes suggestive of the early phases of malignancy. People identified by such nevi need to be examined periodically to ensure that the nevi are not developing into melanoma.

Suspected causes

CHEMICAL AGENTS

Increased risk of melanoma among users of oral contraceptives has been noted in some studies in the order of twofold increase for five or more years of use. However, it cannot be concluded that such exposures are causal, as the studies had not fully explored the effects of recreational sunlight exposure and constitutional factors. Increased risk to melanoma has been suspected as being associated with sunscreen use. Once again, in the several studies that have shown this association, it has been difficult to control for the inevitable increase in sun exposure that tends to accompany sunscreen use, and the fact that those who use sunscreens tend to be those who are constitutionally predisposed to increase risk of melanoma following such exposure.

PHYSICAL AGENTS

Exposure to ultraviolet light in tanning salons increases the risk of melanoma.

Physical trauma to the feet seems to explain the rare acral type of malignant melanoma on the soles of the feet, especially those that occur in Africa.

Unproven causes

PHYSICAL AGENTS

There has been some suspicion that exposure to fluorescent lights at work may increase the risk of melanoma. This is unconfirmed. It seems probable that the excess among people with such exposure may be due to their recreational pursuits, which were not fully evaluated in the studies that resulted in the suspicion of risk from fluorescent light.

DIET

A few studies have suggested a protective effect for melanoma with consumption of vitamin E or beta-carotene.

Prevention

PRIMARY

It is particularly important in those constitutionally predisposed to melanoma (fair skin, susceptibility to burn on exposure to sun) that heavy sun exposure be avoided in childhood. Every measure should be taken to protect such children against sunburn, although with the present uncertainty, no reliance should be placed on sunscreens. Thus young children should play in the shade and wear light-coloured protective clothing.

Such protection should extend throughout life, again with no reliance (according to present evidence) on protection from sunscreens. Thus, the same measures are required as indicated for children: avoiding unprotected exposure to sunlight when the sun is at its peak (solar midday and two to three hours around this), wearing light-coloured protective clothing and broad brimmed hats, and sitting in the shade. In some areas where the population is particularly at risk from melanoma, some radio stations broadcast warnings of anticipated high levels of ambient ultraviolet light exposure at certain times. Such warnings should be heeded, especially by caretakers of young children.

It is not clear whether the gradual acquisition of a tan, without burning, is protective against melanoma. The major difficulty is that those who can acquire a tan have constitutionally a lower risk of melanoma than those who cannot.

SECONDARY (EARLY DETECTION)

As yet, screening for melanoma is not established as effective. However, there is circumstantial evidence that skin inspection on a regular basis—by health professionals, family members, or by oneself—can promote early detection and increase the chance of cure of melanomas. Such approaches are particularly important in those known to be constitutionally predisposed—those who have had severe sun exposure and episodes of burning, and in those with the dysplastic nevus syndrome.

Overall summary

There seems little doubt that the large proportion (90%) of malignant melanomas are caused by ultraviolet light exposure, especially with burning, in those constitutionally predisposed. Perhaps not more than 5% of melanomas in a population are due to sunlight exposure among those with the dysplastic nevus syndrome.

Chapter 24

Other Skin Cancers

In this chapter I consider all cancers of the skin except malignant melanoma, described in the chapter preceding this one, Kaposi's sarcoma, and cancers affecting two special areas adjacent to normal skin: cancers of the lip, and cancers of the anogenital region. The latter, at least in women, have some resemblance to cancers of the vulva, and have been included there.

Kaposi's sarcoma is a special form of cancer affecting the skin that used to be very rare, but which is now occurring in many populations because of the AIDS epidemic. It is now known to be caused by a special virus (human herpes virus type 8) in HIV-infected individuals and it will not be further considered in this chapter.

The skin consists of a stratified squamous epithelium lying on a fibrous layer called the dermis. The epithelium of the skin is constantly renewing itself, with cells multiplying in the basal layer just above the dermis. As these cells get nearer the surface they become horny, or acquire keratin, and become very thin, but form a protective layer against damage and environmental insults. In most of the skin there are varying numbers of hairs. The base or follicle of the hair is where the hair grows. The epithelium that produces the hair is in fact an extension of that on the surface of the skin.

There are two principal types of skin cancers—basal-cell and squamous-cell. Basal-cell cancers are relatively indolent, often pearly white in colour, grow slowly locally, often seem to develop from hair follicles, and can invade surrounding tissue but do not metastasise. Squamous-cell cancers behave like any other malignancy; however, they can metastasise (usually first to local lymph nodes) as well as invade locally. In squamous-cell skin cancers necrosis can occur in the centre, so the cancer may appear as a small ulcer, with heaped up tissue around the edges. The distinction between these two forms of skin cancer can usually be made clinically, but readily by a pathologist if a biopsy is taken or if an excised specimen is sent to pathology.Because basal- and squamous-cell skin cancers are usually easily detected they tend to come to medical attention fairly promptly and are therefore diagnosed early. Those diagnosed are usually treated as outpatients in the offices of skin specialists or dermatologists. The specimens are often not sent to a pathology laboratory and tend not to be recorded in cancer registries; hence, unless the registry makes a special effort to record them, incidence data are often simply not available. This paucity of data makes it difficult to provide as much descriptive information as for most other cancers.

Nevertheless, some estimates have been made of the frequency of skin cancers, and they usually result, at least in fair-skinned populations, in the conclusion that skin cancer is the most common form of all cancers in both sexes combined. In Canada, for example, using the data from one cancer registry with good data collection procedures for skin cancer, it was estimated that 34% of all cancers that were diagnosed in the year 2000 were non-melanoma skin cancers.

The incidence of other skin cancers (basal- and squamous-cell combined) increases by age, with similar rates in males and females at younger ages, and higher rates in males than females at older ages. The rates are much higher (indeed, the highest recorded in the world) in Europeans living in Zimbabwe Africa than in people of similar ancestry living in England and Wales. Rates are very low in Africans in Zimbabwe and also in Japanese, but again, rates are higher at older ages.

Everywhere in the world the incidence of skin cancer is substantially higher than mortality, while incidence is much higher in European countries and Australasia than in countries such as Japan and Hong Kong and is higher in males than females. However, this difference between males and females is substantially less than the difference between Europe and Asia.

There are some data that suggest that incidence has been increasing in Canada and Europe (except possibly for females in Spain), but hardly at all in Asia.In some countries, especially in recent years, there has been an increase in skin cancer mortality. Although this may reflect the increases in incidence also occurring in these countries, there is a possibility that deaths from Kaposi's sarcoma are being wrongly certified to other skin cancers and that the mortality from other skin cancers is in fact stable.

Survival from skin cancers is good; it is unusual for someone with basal-cell carcinoma of the skin to die from the consequences of the cancer—it would have to had been neglected by the patient for a very long time for it to have extended far enough locally to result in death.

Thus, the few deaths that occur are almost invariably due to squamous-cell skin cancers, but even for them recorded survival exceeds 95%.

For squamous-cell skin cancers, a recognised precursor is actinic keratosis, a sun-induced change in the skin that may eventually change to invasive cancer. Actinic keratoses are premalignant lesions characterized by keratinized patches with aberrant cell differentiation and proliferation.

There is no known precursor for basal-cell carcinoma that is recognised clinically, although actinic keratoses probably represent risk factors for basal-cell carcinoma.

Proven causes of skin cancer

PHYSICAL AGENTS

The principal cause of both forms of skin cancer is exposure to the sun. In contradistinction to malignant melanoma of the skin, both basal- and squamous-cell skin cancers occur predominantly on skin normally exposed to the sun. Further, the greater the cumulative sun exposure, the greater the risk of developing skin cancer. That is why skin cancers occur most commonly in the old, and also tend to be more frequent in workers who spend a great deal of time in the sun than in those who work indoors.

CHEMICAL AGENTS

Exposure to arsenic through occupation, medicinal use, or, in some populations, drinking water contamination from dumps or natural arsenic deposits has been found to increase skin cancer risk.

Similarly, exposure to coal tar pitches, largely through road working, roofing, and coal gasification, has also been found to induce skin cancers in those occupationally exposed.

The chemical 8-methylpsoralen is occasionally used as a medication for severe psoriasis. Unfortunately, when treated skin is exposed to ultraviolet radiation, the carcinogenic effect of the sun's ultra violet rays on the skin is enhanced, and skin cancers can result.

Exposure of the skin of the scrotum in young boys to the soot from chimneys was the first occupational cause of skin cancer, identified in the 18th century in Great Britain by surgeon Percival Pott. Scrotal cancers in workers have also occurred as a result of clothing becoming saturated with shale oils used as cutting oils and from exposure to coal tar and coal gasification.

GENETIC SUSCEPTIBILITY

People with fair skin and hair are constitutionally at greater risk of skin cancer than those with dark skin. This is exhibited by the markedly different incidence of skin cancer in different countries, with much greater risk in northern Europe and North America and much less risk in native Africans and Asians.

FAMILIAL CANCER SYNDROMES

A rare inherited abnormality, xeroderma pigmentosum, results in the individual being markedly susceptible to the effect of ultra violet radiation with a substantial risk of skin cancer, often over all sun-exposed sites and commencing in childhood. Only very strict avoidance of sun exposure is able to prevent this.

Suspected causes

CHEMICAL AGENTS

Exposure to creosotes, and occupational exposures in petroleum refining have been suspected as increasing the risk of skin cancers.

CHRONIC INFECTIONS

There is increasing evidence that some forms of skin cancer are caused by specific strains of HPV (the wart virus).

Prevention

PRIMARY

Primary prevention of skin cancer is principally through avoidance of excessive exposure to sun. Sunscreens are probably protective against squamous-cell skin cancers, but there is doubt that they are protective against basal-cell carcinomas. As for melanoma of the skin, there is room for concern that over-reliance on sunscreens could increase sun exposure and enhance carcinogenicity. Therefore use of sunscreens should not be regarded as a justification to increase exposure to ultraviolet light; rather, they should be judicially used in conjunction with appropriate protective clothing.

SECONDARY (EARLY DETECTION)

Screening for skin cancer is not generally advocated. However, awareness of the possibility of skin cancer development is important, especially in the elderly or in those known to have had prolonged exposure to sunlight. Thus, early consultation with a dermatologist is recommended if a suspicious lesion develops.

Overall summary

Probably at least 80% of the skin cancers that occur are explained by exposure to sunlight.

Chapter 25

Bone Cancers

Cancers can occur in any bone, but tend to be more common in the long bones. The bone cancers considered in this chapter are primary—that is, they arise from the tissues of the bone itself and are to be distinguished from the metastases, or secondary deposits, from other cancers such as of the lung, breast, or prostate that have spread to the bone through the bloodstream. The term also excludes those cancers that arise primarily from the bone marrow, such as deposits of multiple myeloma, considered in a separate chapter.

Bone is formed by special cells called osteocytes and continually remodelled with growth and development by other cells called osteoclasts. The osteocytes lay down bone, a calcified mineral, within a fibrous tissue structure. These cells are not epithelial cells that form the lining of an organ, or glandular cells that form structures that secrete substances into their lumen, but a class called mesenchymal cells. If such cells become cancerous, the type of cancer formed is called a sarcoma, and not a carcinoma. The common type of bone cancer is therefore called an osteosarcoma. Other types of bone cancers include chondrosarcomas (believed to arise from the cartilage at the ends of bones), fibrosarcomas, malignant fibrous histiocytomas, and angiosarcomas (so called because of their vascular nature). In children a special type of bone cancer occurs (as do osteosarcomas) called Ewing's sarcoma. Approximately 30% of bone tumours are osteosarcomas, 20% chondrosarcomas, 12% Ewing's sarcoma, and the remainder other groups or are unspecified as to histology.

At all ages incidence rates tend to be higher in males than in females, but differences are not great, while there are remarkable similarities in the rates in the different registries. The rates are low; a cumulative rate to age 74, equivalent to lifetime risk, does not exceed 2 per 1,000 in any registry with reliable data, and a normal rate of about 1 per 1,000 in most countries in males and fewer in females. Mortality data are not readily available but are probably not dissimilar.Unusual compared to other cancers are the relatively high rates for children around ages 5-15. This creates a peak at these ages, and similarly elevated rates do not occur until older ages in adults, although they then rise to higher levels, especially in males; the risk per individual child is low.

Data from cancer registries from countries with long-running cancer registration show no major changes in bone cancer incidence with time for either males or females. International data for trends in mortality are not available.

Survival from bone cancer varies by histological type. In the US, the five-year survival for males with osteosarcoma is approximately 45%, for chondrosarcoma 68%, and 40% for Ewing's sarcoma. The corresponding proportions for females are 61%, 74%, and 55%, respectively. In Europe data are available for all types of bone cancer combined. At all ages the five-year survival for all ages is about 45%, slightly less in males than females. Survival varies by age, however, ranging from around 56% at ages 20-44 falling to under 20% at 75 or older. Data are sparse from developing countries, but in Shanghai five-year survival is just under 20% in both sexes.

No known precursors of bone cancer are recognised. However, the increase in rates of bone cancer coincides with the adolescent bone growth spurt. In adults there is a strong association of osteosarcoma with a degenerative change in bone called Paget's disease; the pathogenesis, is however, unknown.

Proven causes of bone cancers

CHEMICAL AGENTS

There are associations between use of alkylating agents for the treatment of childhood cancers and the subsequent development of bone cancer in the same children.

PHYSICAL AGENTS

Radiation in different forms is known to increase the risk of bone cancer. The classic studies related to people exposed to radium, especially to glow-in-the-dark paints used on the dials of aircraft instruments in the early years of the 20th century. The workers, mostly women, used to point the brush with their lips, leading to the ingestion of small amounts of radium-containing paste. The radium was deposited in bone and osteosarcomas subsequently developed in a high proportion of those exposed, often after many years. Other exposure to radium, such as the injection of radium for treatment of some illnesses, has also been shown to increase the risk of bone cancer.

There are no known lifestyle determinants of bone cancer.

Genetic susceptibility

FAMILIAL CANCER SYNDROMES

Bone cancer is increased in Li-Fraumeni syndrome. This is a rare syndrome that occurs in families and is known to be associated with a mutation of the p53 cancer suppressor gene. Other cancers increased in these families include soft-tissue sarcomas, cancers of the breast, brain, adrenals, and leukemia.

MULTIGENIC SUSCEPTIBILITY

There is an association between genetic susceptibility to retino-blastomas and increased risk of osteogenic sarcomas. This may be due to another gene acting in concert with the retinoblastoma gene, which increases the risk of tumours of the retina of the eye.

Suspected causes

PHYSICAL AGENTS

RADIATION

"Bone-seeking" radioactive isotopes other than radium may also increase the risk of bone cancer, such as caesium and thorium released in radioactive fallout after atomic bomb explosions in the atmosphere, and in the case of caesium, in the Chernobyl nuclear plant exposure. However, in the latter instance, it is not yet known whether there will be an increase in bone cancer in the exposed populations.

Prevention

PRIMARY

The only known preventive action possible for bone tumours is reduction in exposure to radiation. In practice, people are no longer exposed to the known radiation related exposures that increased the risk of bone cancer.

SECONDARY (EARLY DETECTION)

There is no screening test for bone cancer.

Overall summary

Currently, the proportion of bone cancers explained by the various known risk factors is extremely small.

Chapter 26

Connective Tissue Cancers

Connective tissue is present throughout the body, within and between all organs. When cooks prepare meat, the connective tissue is the layer of fibrous material between the muscles that they usually cut out. Within organs, the blood vessels, glandular structures, etc., all are supported by a connective tissue called stroma. The principal cells that produce this stroma are called fibroblasts.

When cancer develops in connective tissue, with malignant transformation of fibroblasts and sometimes of other lining cells of glands and blood vessels (endothelial cells), the type of cancer that develops is called a sarcoma, rather than a carcinoma. The term "soft tissue sarcoma" is often applied to this group of cancers.

The different names given to types of connective tissue sarcomas include fibrosarcomas, malignant fibrous histiocytomas, angiosarcomas, malignant giant cell tumours, and unspecified sarcomas. The fibrosarcomas, which are the commonest, arise from normal supportive connective tissue; angiosarcomas, as their name implies, are vascular tumours believed to arise from blood vessels. These largely occur in the extremities. In addition, leiomyosarcomas of the uterus and gastro-intestinal tract occur principally in adults, and liposarcomas in the extremities and trunk. Rhabdomyosarcomas occur in the head, neck, and in the genito-urinary tract. In children rhabdo-myosarcomas occur in the extremities; these are the most common forms of childhood connective tissue tumours. They occur in very young children, hence they often carry the designation embryonal.

Although cancers of connective tissue can occur at any age, they are far more frequent in adults than children and their frequency increases progressively throughout life. In adults rates are higher in males than females.

While these sarcomas are, in practice, more frequent in adults than the other group of sarcomas occurring in bone, in children bone tumours are more frequent than connective tissue tumours, although bone tumours tend to occur in older children.

There are not large differences in the incidence of cancers of connective worldwide. Incidence is lower in Japan than the West and in China and other parts of Asia incidence is intermediary. In the US mortality from cancers of connective tissue has been increasing, although at least some of this is due to the increase in Kaposi's sarcoma, the cancer linked with AIDS. Over time, the tendency has been for incidence to increase or remain stable. In North America and Europe the five-year survival of cancers of connective tissue approximates to 50% in both males and females. In most developing countries survival is much lower—no more than 30%.

Proven causes of connective tissue cancers

CHEMICAL AGENTS

Occupational exposure to vinyl chloride has been shown to increase the risk of angiosarcomas of the liver.

Angiosarcomas of the liver have also followed the prolonged use of arsenic-containing medicaments.

Sarcomas can occur at the site of injections of a persistent iron-containing preparation such as iron-dextran, used to treat iron-deficiency anemia.

PHYSICAL AGENTS

A small proportion of cancers of connective tissue occur following intense radiation exposure.

CHRONIC INFECTIONS

While a virus causes Kaposi's sarcoma, viruses have not been linked to other cancers of connective tissue.

Genetic susceptibility

FAMILIAL CANCER SYNDROMES

Cancers of connective tissue are increased in Li-Fraumeni syndrome. Other cancers increased in these families include osteogenic sarcomas, cancers of the breast, brain, adrenals, and leukemia.

Neurofibrosarcomas also occur in the congenital genetic disorder neurofibromatosis syndrome.

There is an association between genetic susceptibility to retinoblastomas and increased risk of connective tissue sarcomas in survivors of retinoblastoma. This may well be due to another gene acting in concert with the retinoblastoma gene, which increases the risk of tumours of the retina of the eye.

Suspected causes

CHEMICAL AGENTS

Occupations involving exposure to herbicides, some pesticides, and chlorophenols have been strongly suspected as increasing the risk of cancers of connective tissue.

Exposure to Agent Orange, a herbicide used extensively in military campaigns in Southeast Asia, has also been suspected as increasing the risk of connective tissue sarcomas.

Prevention

PRIMARY

Reduction in exposure to herbicides and pesticides may reduce the risk of these cancers.

SECONDARY (EARLY DETECTION)

There is no known screening test for cancers of connective tissue.

Overall summary

Connective tissue cancers are relatively rare. The proportion of connective tissue sarcomas that can be explained by known risk factors is small.

Chapter 27

Cancers of the Eye

The eye is an unusual site for cancers as it is a complex structure, perfectly designed for vision but with most of its contents (including the cornea, lens, and vitreous humour behind the lens) non-cellular, therefore unable to develop into cancers. However, some cancers do arise within the eye in some of its components, especially the conjunctival lining of the eye, the iris, and the light-receiving retina at the back of the eye, essentially an extension of the optic nerve, itself an extension of the brain.

The cancers that arise within the eye complex include epidermoid cancers of the conjunctiva and cornea, melanomas of the iris, retinoblastomas arising within the retina, adenocarcinomas of the lachrymal gland and duct, lymphomas of the orbit, soft-part sarcomas of the orbit, and some unspecified cancers.

However, eye cancers are rare in both males and females. The majority of eye cancers in adults are melanomas, which make up about three-quarters of eye cancers in Western populations, and the majority of eye cancers in children are retinoblastomas, which occur mainly in the first years of life and comprise about 15% of eye cancers. For more information on retinoblastomas see the chapter on cancers in children.

The frequency of occurrence of eye cancers is higher in Western countries than in Asia. There is a high rate in Australia, due to eye melanomas occurring in a susceptible population of Western origin.

Melanoma of the eye has increased in recent years, in parallel with melanoma of the skin, presumably due to increasing exposure to ultraviolet light by those susceptible.

Survival is good in those in whom eye cancers are found to be still confined to the eye.

Proven causes of eye cancers

PHYSICAL AGENTS

Melanomas of the eye, as for melanomas of the skin, are believed to be due to exposure to ultraviolet light especially in blue-eyed, fair-skinned people.

Genetic susceptibility

FAMILIAL CANCER SYNDROMES

Retinoblastoma has a genetic component, as discussed in the chapter on childhood cancers.

Prevention

PRIMARY

For melanomas of the eye the only known preventive maneuver is reduction in exposure to ultraviolet light by wearing UV-absorbent sunglasses.

Chapter 28

Central Nervous System (Brain) Cancers

The most important tumours of the central nervous system arise in the brain or its coverings. There are two types of brain tumour: tumours affecting the lining of the brain, the meninges (called meningiomas, which are usually benign), and cancers that develop in the supporting tissue within the brain itself. Tumours that can develop in the lining of nerves comprise less than 10% of central nervous system tumours. The majority of these develop in the lining surrounding the auditory nerve, the nerve from the ear to the brain, and are called auditory neuromas.

Brain cancer can occur in children and adults, although the types of cancers that occur in children tend to be different than those that occur in adults; the term malignant embryonal tumours is used to describe them, including medulloblastomas, which originate toward the posterior aspect of the brain and tend to affect children more frequently than adults. Brain cancers derived from the supporting tissue within the brain are largely derived from cells called astrocytes (hence the term astrocytoma) or the glial cells (glioblastoma) and are cancers that tend to be highly malignant and usually fatal. Brain cancers may be classified according to the area of the brain in which they arise and thus there are frontal tumours, temporal lobe tumours, and tumours of the cerebellum.

There is a small peak of incidence of brain tumours in young children, then a rise in incidence that continues throughout life. The incidence of brain cancer is higher in men than in women.

There is about a fourfold difference in incidence of brain tumours between technically advanced and developing countries, although it is likely that poor ascertainment of brain tumours accounts for at least some of the low incidence in developing countries.

In technically advanced countries the incidence of brain cancer was increasing until about two decades ago. Much of this was regarded as due to improvements in imaging methods, including brain CTs (computerized tomography), especially distinguishing them from strokes when they bleed internally. Since then, in most countries, incidence of brain cancers has remained stable, although the rates are still increasing in some middle-income countries.

Survival is low for the most malignant tumours (glioblastomas)—very few survive more than five years. In contrast, patients with meningioma have very good survival, provided diagnosis is prompt. Patients with nerve sheath tumours also survive well.

Gliomas differ in grade, a difference correlated with survival. It is suspected that low-grade gliomas can evolve into high-grade gliomas, facilitated by genetic mutations.

Proven causes of cancers of the nervous system

PHYSICAL AGENTS

Ionising radiation (such as low-dose radiation for treatment of fungal infections of the scalp, a past practice that is now strongly discouraged), if directed to the brain, will increase the risk of brain cancer.

Genetic susceptibility

FAMILIAL CANCER SYNDROMES

Some brain tumours are associated with inherited cancer syndromes—such as Li-Fraumeni, Cowden, and Turcot syndromes—but they are rare, as is a family history of brain cancer. Genetic changes have been found in many brain cancers, but these are probably acquired during tumour development and are not inherited.

Suspected causes

CHEMICAL AGENTS

Some studies have suggested increased risk of brain cancers in certain occupations, including firefighters and those working in the petroleum refining industry. Specific causal agents have not been identified, however.

PHYSICAL AGENTS

Non-ionising radiation, especially electric and magnetic fields, have been suspected to increase the risk of brain cancers in workers who were heavily exposed to electric fields, such as workers in the electric generation and transmission industry.

Of greater concern has been the increasing evidence that the radiofrequency field exposure inherent in the use of mobile phones and Wi-Fi, especially by children, will increase the risk of brain cancer. In adults there is some evidence of a dose response for risk of brain cancers in those with longest exposure and greatest use of mobile phones; the brain cancers that occurred were localized in the areas of maximum exposure in the brain. There have also been some studies suggesting that such exposure increases the risk of auditory neuromas and salivary gland tumours.

DIET

There has been some suspicion that nitrosamines formed from exposure to high levels of nitrite in some preserved foods could increase the risk of brain cancer in humans because such an effect has been found in experimental animals. In general, heavily nitrosated foods should be avoided as they increase the risk of stomach cancer, and, in the form of preserved meats, colon cancer. The evidence that they increase the risk of brain cancer, however, is uncertain.

Prevention

The only known action that will prevent brain cancers is avoidance of radiation to the brain.

However, many now advocate the precautionary principle, seeking reduction of exposure to radiofrequency fields (Wi-Fi), and devices that depend upon them, including smart meters and mobile phones. Thus, hands-free devices are encouraged for mobile phone use, and especially, reduction of exposure to mobile phones in children and young adults as their brains are believed to be more sensitive to the effects of radiofrequency fields than those of adults. Manufacturers of cell phones include a warning that the phones should be kept away from the body, especially when in use, but this is often printed in small print and tends to be ignored.

Some governments have issued an advisory urging that exposure of children to mobile phones should be reduced.

Overall summary

Other than the rare family syndromes known to be associated with brain cancer, the etiology of brain cancers is uncertain, apart from the small proportion caused by ionising radiation. However, there is increasing concern that radiofrequency fields associated with mobile phone use may increase the risk of brain cancer and also some suggestions that dietary factors may play a role.

Chapter 29

Thyroid Cancer

The thyroid is an endocrine gland—one of those glands that secrete hormones into the bloodstream to control body metabolism. It is situated in the neck near the trachea, just below the larynx. It has a lateral lobe on each side and a connecting "bridge"—the isthmus of the thyroid. Its function is to secrete thyroxine into the blood. When the gland is chronically overactive, the state of hyperthyroidism occurs, diagnosed because of a tendency for the eyes to protrude (exophthalmos), the thyroid to swell, the patient to lose weight and to feel hot, and to be in a state of overactivity. Hyperthyroidism tends to increase the risk of thyroid cancer developing. When the thyroid gland's function is subnormal the patient is lethargic, the skin becomes waxy and the face puffy, and the patient tends to feel cold, a condition called myxoedema. The thyroid gland requires an adequate supply of iodine in the diet to produce thyroxine. If iodine is deficient, as in some mountainous areas in Europe such as Switzerland, the thyroid gland swells and a goiter develops. If this condition develops in childhood, mental deficiency supervenes and the child develops pinched features and is called cretinous or a cretin. The gland can also be affected with a form of inflammation called thyroiditis.

The thyroid is not a common site of cancer. It has been estimated in the US, for example, that thyroid cancer comprises only about 0.5% of cancers in males and 1.7% of cancers in females.

As the thyroid is a glandular organ, the cancers that occur are almost invariably carcinomas. They are classified according to their appearance on microscopy; 58% are papillary carcinomas, 17% follicular, and the remainder of various types, including medullary carcinomas.

The rates of thyroid cancer are universally higher in females than males, a well-recognised feature of this cancer, and higher in North America than in the UK. The age distribution for Canada and the US is different from many other cancers, with higher rates at younger ages.

There is substantial variation in rates of incidence of thyroid cancer worldwide, with the highest rates in North America and the lowest in Asia. Mortality does not vary as much, with mortality in females in North America being less than that in other regions. Rates for males show similar differences, but at lower levels.

Internationally, the general trend in incidence in both men and women is upwards. It is suspected that increase in diagnostic activity may in part be responsible, and that some of the cancers detected may be over-diagnosed, in other words, they would not have presented in the patient in their lifetime in the absence of the diagnostic test.

Survival from thyroid cancer is excellent, with relative survival rates (the survival from the cancer relative to the expected survival of people free of the cancer and of the same age and sex) approximating to 95%. In Canada, the five-year relative survival for thyroid cancer increased from 93% in 1992-94 to 98% in 2005-07.

There are different histological types of thyroid cancer; papillary and follicular predominate. Papillary thyroid cancer has the best prognosis and survival is excellent. Follicular cancer also has a good prognosis, except when metastases are present. Therefore, although there has been concern that modern methods of diagnosis may over-diagnose thyroid cancer, once the presence of the cancer is confirmed, prompt treatment is recommended to avoid the development of metastases.

Proven causes of thyroid cancer

PHYSICAL AGENTS

Ionising radiation is known to increase the risk of thyroid cancer, especially papillary cancer. In the past, radiation was used for the treatment of benign conditions, even tinea capitis, a fungal infection of the scalp. Such radiation has been shown to increase the risk of thyroid cancer. Radioactive iodine has been used in the past for many diagnostic purposes, especially diagnosis of thyroid-related diseases. As the radioactive iodine is concentrated in the thyroid, there is reason to be somewhat concerned. Indeed, such usage has been demonstrated to double the risk of subsequent thyroid cancer. Such use should no longer be of concern given that radioactive iodine has effectively been replaced by the use of other diagnostic methods.

Radioactive iodine was released to the environment during the Chernobyl nuclear disaster and a release was also associated with the experimental Hanford reactor in the US. Within a few years those exposed were found to have an increased risk of thyroid cancer, an excess that was also seen in neighbouring countries to the Ukraine that were exposed to the radioactive cloud released into the atmosphere by the explosion of the Chernobyl nuclear reactor. A similar but lesser effect occurred following the Fukishima nuclear plant disaster in Japan. However, some of these increases may be artifactual, caused by the application of tests that found areas interpreted as cancer but which were not progressive (over-diagnosis).

DIET

Iodine-deficient diets, such as those of areas where goitre occurs are known to be associated with an increased risk of thyroid cancer.

FAMILIAL CANCER SYNDROMES

About 20% of one form of thyroid cancer, the medullary form, appears to have a familial origin. This can occur alone or as part of a multiple endocrine neoplasia (MEN) syndrome. A small proportion of papillary thyroid cancers have been associated with familial polyposis coli.

Suspected causes

DIET

A protective effect of cruciferous vegetables has been suggested as well as an increased risk with consumption of certain sea foods.

REPRODUCTIVE BEHAVIOUR

A weak association between both parity and miscarriage and thyroid cancer has been found in a few studies.

Prevention

PRIMARY

Iodine tablets should be consumed by those exposed to excess radioactivity or radioiodine to prevent the uptake of radioiodine by the thyroid.

SECONDARY (EARLY DETECTION)

As the thyroid is a superficial organ, early detection simply takes the form of evaluating any nodules that newly appear.

Overall Summary

The proportion of thyroid cancers explained by the various risk factors cannot yet be determined.

Chapter 30

Hodgkin Disease

Hodgkin disease is a malignancy of the immune system and is a form of the type of cancer called lymphomas. It affects young people and adults, and the shape of the incidence curve is bimodal, with a peak in young adulthood and another peak in later adult years. It was named after Thomas Hodgkin, who first described abnormalities in the lymph system in 1832. It is not a common cancer—in North America it amounts to about 1% of all cancer cases.

The clinical and histologic features of Hodgkin disease suggest an infectious process. The disease is characterized by the orderly spread of disease from one lymph node group to another, often first detected in the neck or axilla, and then by the development of systemic symptoms with advanced disease. Patients with systemic symptoms tend to have an enlarged spleen and sometimes an enlarged liver. Other nodes in the body, the groin, for example, the mediastinum (middle of the chest), or abdomen may be found to be involved by the disease. When Hodgkin cells are examined microscopically, multinucleated Reed-Sternberg cells (RS cells) are the characteristic histopathologic finding. Based on histological features, the disease may be classified into four major categories:

lymphocyte predominance, nodular sclerosis, mixed cellularity, and lymphocyte depletion.

Hodgkin disease is more common in men than in women, especially at older ages. The age distribution is very different from the more common carcinomas such as those of the breast, colon, lung, or prostate, with the early peak in incidence around age 20-25, and then a fall in incidence, with a much greater age peak at ages 70-80. It is the early age peak that is so atypical.

The highest rates of Hodgkin disease are reported from North America and Europe, the lowest from India and Japan. The overall five-year relative survival for 2001–2007 from 17 geographic areas in the US was 83.9%. Since many patients are young, they often live 40 years or more after treatment. This relatively high survival indicates the success of modern treatment for this disease—radiotherapy and then combination regimens of chemotherapy.

Proven causes of Hodgkin disease

CHRONIC INFECTIONS

There is a great deal of evidence linking Hodgkin disease to infection with the Epstein-Barr virus. This virus is the cause of a common disease (infectious mononucleosis), associated with changes in immune cells. Hodgkin disease, especially in younger people, seems to be due to an atypical infection with the virus, possibly due to individual susceptibility by causes not yet recognized.

Suspected causes

CHEMICAL AGENTS

There is some evidence that Hodgkin disease is increased in workers in wood-related occupations. The causal factor has not been identified.

CHRONIC INFECTIONS

A number of investigations have suggested that Hodgkin disease may be caused by several not yet identified infectious agents other than the Epstein-Barr virus. Some studies have suggested a type of transmission from case to case—a "clustering" of cases, —giving support to the infectious agent or agents causal hypothesis.

Prevention

PRIMARY

No preventive approach has yet been identified.

Overall summary

Hodgkin disease is relatively rare. It occurs in young people (teenage to early adult years) with another peak in the elderly. It appears to be the result of a disturbance of the immune system following atypical infection with the ubiquitous Epstein-Barr virus. Modern treatment results in high survival.

Chapter 31

Non-Hodgkin Lymphomas

The non-Hodgkin lymphomas are a group of cancers affecting the immune system that do not have the characteristics of Hodgkin disease. They can be generalized or affect a specific organ, for example, a lymphoma of the stomach. Because of their heterogeneous nature, it is important that they be fully characterised, both to begin to understand their causes and origin and the preferred treatment.

Since they were first recognised as an entity the non-Hodgkin lymphomas have undergone a series of changes in pathologic classification. Now, they are generally classified by their presumed cell of origin—B-cell lymphoma—as well as whether the disease is generalised or appears to be localised to a specific organ. In the past, the terms used were reticulum cell sarcoma and lymphosarcoma, then these were replaced by a classification based on the descriptive nature of the tissues affected—diffuse lymphocytic or histiocytic, nodular diffuse, or histiocytic. Also, these types were subdivided into the degree of differentiation of the cells. Thus, the B-cell lymphomas may be distinguished as low-grade or high-grade and distinguished from the T-cell lymphomas. One specific type of lymphoma with special characteristics, first recognised in East

Africa by surgeon Denis Burkitt, is called Burkitt's lymphoma. Apart from Burkitt's lymphoma, most studies of the etiology of the lymphomas have not distinguished the specific sub-types, but instead considered them as a group, a situation that also occurs in incidence and mortality statistics.

The incidence of non-Hodgkin lymphomas increases progressively throughout life, with the highest incidence at ages 80-84. Incidence is greater in men than women. Although overall the incidence of the lymphomas is nearly 10 times that of Hodgkin disease, the incidence at younger ages is so low that the incidence of Hodgkin disease is much higher than of the non-Hodgkin lymphomas up to the age of 25.

There is substantial variation in incidence of the non-Hodgkin lymphomas internationally, with the rates highest in North America, Europe, and Australasia, and lowest in India and China. In each country, rates are higher in men than women.

There have been major increases in the incidence of non-Hodgkin lymphoma in both males and females. These increases have occurred in all countries studied. One reason for these increases is the association of the AIDS with the development of lymphomas. (See chronic infections, below.) Another reason could be the link with some chemicals that accumulate in the environment, especially pesticides and herbicides. (See suspected causes, chemical agents, below.) However, it is generally accepted that we do not have a satisfactory explanation for much of the increase in incidence and that research to try and understand the cause or causes of the increase is desirable.

Patients with low-grade tumours have relatively good survival and those with high-grade (diffuse) tumours have a poor survival. Survival has improved with modern chemotherapy regimens, but not to a great extent.

Proven causes of the lymphomas

RADIATION

Studies of patients who received spinal irradiation for the treatment of ankylosing spondylitis showed an increased risk of non-Hodgkin lymphoma. However, in other irradiated populations (including atomic bomb survivors), no increased incidence of lymphoma was found.

CHRONIC INFECTIONS

Burkitt's lymphoma in Africa has been linked to infection with the Epstein-Barr virus, superimposed on a disturbance of the immune system caused by hyperimmunity to malaria.

Another infectious disease link with a different form of lymphoma is the association of Kaposi's sarcoma with AIDS. In people with AIDS, Kaposi's sarcoma is caused by an interaction between HIV (the virus that causes AIDS), a weakened immune system (the consequence of AIDS), and another virus, the human herpesvirus-8 (HHV-8). Kaposi's sarcoma is thus linked to the spread of HIV and HHV-8 through sexual activity.

DISTURBANCE WITH IMMUNE MECHANISMS

Non-Hodgkin lymphomas occur with increased frequency in persons who are receiving immune suppressing drugs because of transplant surgery, commonly following bone or renal transplants.

Suspected causes

RADIATION

In one study of workers occupationally exposed to high levels of electrical fields there was a significant increase in the risk of lymphomas.

CHEMICAL AGENTS

There has been suspicion for some time that one of the reasons for the increase in incidence of the lymphomas was the entry of various chemicals into the environment. Of particular concern was the accumulation in the environment of various pesticides and herbicides. It would not be surprising if these chemicals, developed to kill living organisms, also affected mankind; indeed, there is no question that the majority of these chemicals in high dosage will cause acute neurological or other effects. A particular group that might be expected to show effects are pesticide applicators and agricultural workers. Studies of these occupational groups have not yielded entirely consistent results, but there does seem to be an emerging consensus that those who are heavily exposed have an increased risk of lymphoma. Whether that increased risk extends to the general population is unknown.

DIET

No dietary factors have been linked to non-Hodgkin lymphoma.

Genetic susceptibility

FAMILIAL CANCER SYNDROMES

Some associations of lymphomas within families have been reported. However, no specific familial cancer syndrome has been identified, nor have lymphomas been linked to specific genes.

Prevention

PRIMARY

Prevention of transmission of HIV will reduce the incidence of AIDS-associated lymphomas.

It is possible that reducing exposure to pesticides and to high levels of electrical fields will prevent some cases of lymphoma developing.

Overall summary

The non-Hodgkin lymphomas are a heterogeneous group of cancers of the immune system. Some are clearly linked to infection with known viruses; there is a suspicion that some are due to chemical exposures, especially to pesticides, and possibly to high levels of electrical fields.

No quantitative estimate of the effects of such preventive actions is possible at this time.

Chapter 32

The Leukemias

The leukemias are malignancies of the blood-forming tissue, and thus arise in the bone marrow. They are a form of cancer, but are neither carcinomas nor sarcomas. Because the proliferation of leukemic cells tends to displace other blood cells, they may present with the symptoms of anemia or of infection. Thus, the symptoms they give rise to are non-specific and they tend only to be diagnosed when a blood test is done and abnormalities are discovered in the test.

There are four major leukemia cell-type groupings: acute lymphoblastic leukemia, chronic lymphocytic leukemia, acute myeloid leukemia (also called acute non-lymphoblastic leukemia), and chronic myeloid leukemia. Some now regard chronic lymphocytic leukemia as a form of lymphoma.

Two forms of acute leukemia occur in both children and adults—acute lymphocytic and acute myeloid leukemia, acute lymphocytic leukemia being the commonest childhood cancer, although it comprises only about 5% of leukemia in adults age 40 or more. The other forms of leukemia increase in incidence with increasing age, all are more common in men than women.

There is not much variation in leukemia incidence rates world-wide, although they do tend to be recognized more in technically advanced countries, especially chronic lymphocytic leukemia.

As a result of improvements in therapy, especially for childhood leukemia, there have been major falls in mortality from the acute leukemias, especially acute lymphocytic leukemia, in the last few decades. There has also been some reduction in mortality from adult leukemia, again because of improved treatment.

Care needs to be taken in interpreting apparent increases in leukemia in some countries because many of these coincided with increased diagnostic efficiency in recognising the causes of anaemia or unusual infections.

Survival from childhood leukemia now amounts to approximately 80%. Indeed, the improvement of survival has been so dramatic that major efforts are now being made to reduce the long-term side effects from treatment, such as those that followed cranial irradiation, including disturbance of mental function. In adults, leukemia survival approximates to 40-60%, depending on age and severity of disease.

Proven causes of the leukemias

CHEMICAL AGENTS

Exposure to the solvent benzene increases the risk of leukemia, especially of acute myeloid leukemia. Such exposures have occurred in workers exposed to gasoline or petrol and those exposed to adhesives containing benzene such as shoe and leather workers.

Cigarette smoking is now recognised as increasing the risk of acute myeloid leukemia.

PHYSICAL AGENTS

A major cause of the leukemias, except chronic lymphocytic leukemia, is exposure to ionizing radiation, such as among those exposed to the atomic bombs, nuclear reactors, diagnostic X-rays, and CT scans. Since the recognition of such risks, major efforts are taken to reduce such exposures to the minimum using the ALARA (As Low As Reasonably Achievable) principle.

CHRONIC INFECTIONS

A virus, human T-cell lymphotropic virus type I, has been linked with a rare form of adult leukemia in Japan.

Suspected causes

PHYSICAL AGENTS

Leukemia has been associated with exposure to electrical and magnetic fields, especially electric fields in adults occupationally exposed, and leukemia in children has been linked to magnetic fields. The evidence is sufficiently strong that means should be taken to ensure that buildings and schools are not placed within 50 metres of high-voltage transmission lines or transformers.

CHRONIC INFECTIONS

There has been suspicion for some time that leukemia may be caused by infectious agents, but to date no such cause has been proven, apart from the human T-cell lymphotropic virus.

Kinlen's, or the mixing hypothesis, was postulated to explain a higher rate of leukemia in the areas around the British Sellafield nuclear complex in Cumbria than in other parts of the country. The hypothesis is that mixing of the population, which occurred when people started moving into the area to work at the nuclear facility, resulted in the spreading of a virus that could cause leukemia. The theory was first developed in 1988 by cancer researcher Leo Kinlen and has not been supported by research elsewhere. No specific virus has been implicated.

GENETIC SUSCEPTIBILITY

There is some evidence of familial associations with leukemia. However, specific genetic susceptibility has not been identified.

Prevention

PRIMARY

Avoidance of exposure to benzene and ionizing radiation is critical, while it would be also be prudent to reduce exposure to electrical and magnetic fields. Otherwise, prevention of leukemia is not possible.

SECONDARY PREVENTION

Screening is not recommended for early detection of leukemia.

Overall Summary

The leukemias are relatively rare diseases of blood-forming tissue that occur in both children and adults. Apart from some well-recognised occupational causes and the increased risk of all leukemias (except the chronic lymphocytic form) from radiation exposure, it is not possible to develop an estimate of the proportion of leukemias that are preventable.

Chapter 33

Multiple Myeloma

Multiple myeloma is a relatively rare cancer of specialised cells from the bone marrow (plasma cells) that are responsible for fighting infections. It often gives rise to many symptoms, is usually widespread in the body, and may affect bones, resulting in fractures from minimal injury (pathological fractures). It is usually diagnosed following a blood test that shows specialised monoclonal proteins (in the past called Bence-Jones proteins and now usually referred to as light chain proteins), or by a bone marrow biopsy that shows a tumour made of plasma cells.

Multiple myeloma is a disease largely of older adults; incidence increases rapidly with age and it is more frequent in men than women.

Multiple myeloma is more frequent in technically advanced countries than in developing countries. In the US it is more common in blacks than whites.

Survival from multiple myeloma is relatively poor. In spite of chemotherapy, the disease tends to progress, resulting in bony deformities and eventually death.

Proven causes of multiple myeloma

PHYSICAL AGENTS

Ionising radiation is the only established cause of multiple myeloma, although most cases do not seem to be caused by radiation.

Suspected causes

CHEMICAL AGENTS

There has been suspicion that some chemical agents, where exposure has been caused by occupation or may be present in the external environment, may increase the risk of multiple myeloma, for example, benzene, other solvents, and pesticides. However, because of the rarity of the disease, establishing cause and effect relationships has been difficult.

There has also been suspicion that multiple myeloma could be associated with disturbance of the immune system, even being an autoimmune disease, a disease where the cells responsible for protection against infections produce malfunctioning immune bodies that attack the bodies own cells.

Prevention

PRIMARY

Apart from protection against exposure to ionizing radiation, there is no other known means to prevent multiple myeloma.

Chapter 34

Cancers in Children

Cancer is very rare among children everywhere in the world. In technically advanced countries, only about 1 in 200 of all cancers occur among children younger than 15 years.

Childhood cancers are less often carcinomas than in adults. Nearly all the types of cancers that occur in adults can occur in children, but far less frequently. The commonest types of childhood cancers are leukemia, brain cancer, cancers of the bone, a tumour of the eye called retinoblastoma, and a specific cancer of the kidney called Wilm's tumour. But, very rarely, it is also possible for cancers of the breast, lung, and other organs to occur in children.

It is not the purpose of this chapter to repeat the details given in the chapters on specific cancers. Thus information on childhood leukemia will be found in the chapter on leukemias and information on Wilm's tumour will be found in the chapter on kidney cancer.

Childhood tumours tend to be classified principally according to histology or tissue of origin rather than primary site. The recognised childhood cancer types are: leukemia, lymphomas, central nervous system cancers, sympathetic nervous system cancers, retinoblastoma (of the eye), kidney cancers (Wilm's tumour), liver tumours, bone tumours, soft tissue sarcomas, germ cell tumours, trophoblastic and other gonadal cancers, and carcinomas. One specific subtype is neuroblastoma, a cancerous tumour that occurs in infants and children and develops from nerve tissue in the sympathetic nervous system, the nervous system that controls our essential functions without us being conscious of the action. The relative frequency of the different types of childhood cancer for Canada are leukemia 37%, brain 20%, lymphomas 14%, neuroblastoma 7%, bone 6%, connective tissue 5%, Wilm's tumour 5%, retinoblastoma 3%, liver 2%, and testis 2%. The corresponding percentages for girls are almost identical, although ovarian cancer substitutes for testis, and 2% are thyroid cancers.

The incidence of most childhood cancers is higher in boys than in girls. The risk by age depends on the type of tumour, thus retinoblastoma is more frequent in very young children and leukemia tends to be commoner in younger children, but brain cancers have a more uniform age distribution. Retinoblastomas can be bilateral—these are predominantly of genetic origin and can be present at birth. These may be recognised by a pink spot in the pupil in a child who is having difficulty in seeing. However, retinoblastoma is rare, affecting only about one in 20,000 children.

Childhood cancers tend to be more frequent in developed than developing countries, but this is likely to be more a function of recognition and availability of specialist diagnostic units than real variation. Unilateral retinoblastomas appear to be more frequent in black or African populations than in white.

Because of the higher proportion of children in developing countries than in technically advanced countries, deaths from childhood cancer are more significant in developing countries. It has been estimated that for those under five years of age, deaths from cancer comprise 40% of the deaths worldwide in the least developed countries, but only 1% in industrial countries. From 1990 to 2008 there was a 40% reduction in such deaths in industrial countries, but only a 28% reduction in least developed countries.

Survival from childhood cancers has been improving, especially leukemia, due to improved therapy. Recent data from Canada shows that in the order of 85% of children with cancer will survive to age 15 or more.

Proven causes of childhood cancers

PHYSICAL AGENTS

Childhood leukemia can be caused by in utero irradiation by pelvic X-rays during pregnancy (see chapter on leukemia).

CHRONIC INFECTIONS

Burkitt's lymphoma in children has been causally associated with infection by the Epstein-Barr virus (see chapter on lymphomas).

Suspected causes

CHEMICAL AGENTS

A number of attempts have been made to link the occupation of fathers or of mothers to childhood cancer in their offspring, however, causality of the associations seen has not been established.

PHYSICAL AGENTS

Childhood leukemia has been associated with extremely low-frequency electromagnetic fields (see chapter on leukemia).

CHRONIC INFECTIONS

A number of attempts have been made to link childhood cancers to virus infections, especially for leukemia (see the chapter on leukemia).

GENETIC SUSCEPTIBILITY

The retinoblastoma gene initiates retinoblastoma. The cancer results from the deletion of RB1, a tumour suppressor gene whose job it is to regulate cell growth and keep cells from dividing too rapidly or in an uncontrolled way. In about 60% of cases, the RB1 gene is missing from cells in the retina, and patients are not at risk of passing the disease to their offspring. But for the remaining children, the genetic mutation is present in all the cells of their body. Usually, the mutation arises spontaneously around the time of conception, but in 10% of cases the mutated gene is inherited from a parent. These youngsters often develop tumours in both eyes. And, although retinoblastoma has a high cure rate in developed countries, survivors have an elevated risk of developing another form of cancer later in life. If the child carries only one normal copy of the retinoblastoma gene, he or she is at lifelong risk to develop other cancers at a much higher rate than the general population.

FAMILIAL CANCER SYNDROMES

There have been some rare associations identified of possible familial syndromes and childhood cancer, including familial retinoblastoma, Wilm's tumour, Li-Fraumeni syndrome, and multiple endocrine abnormalities, including thyroid cancer. These seem to account for a very low proportion of childhood cancers. A large proportion of familial retinoblastomas are transmitted through an autosomal dominant gene, the retinoblastoma gene.

Children with Down's syndrome have a higher incidence of leukemia than normal children.

Prevention

PRIMARY

The only established preventive action for childhood cancer is reducing exposure to X-rays in pregnancy.

SECONDARY (EARLY DETECTION)

Screening infants for neuroblastoma has been conclusively shown to lead to an increase in incidence of early-stage neuroblastoma, but no decrease in incidence of advanced-stage disease, or of incidence in children older than one year. Thus, screening increased medical care costs, but failed to reduce the incidence of serious disease. This is one of the first identified instances of over-diagnosis from screening. Screening for neuroblastoma (recommended in the past, especially in Japan) is therefore no longer recommended. No screening tests are available for other childhood cancers.

Chapter 35:

Finale: What can be expected from cancer prevention and screening?

Theoretically, it should be possible to prevent at least 50% of cancer cases and deaths from occurring by applying what we know about causation of cancer, and at least a further 10% of cancer deaths by screening. Yet, we seem unable to attain this, although remarkable success has been achieved by preventing smoking-attributable cancers from occurring. The success in reducing smoking was largely due to the application of a fiscal weapon—taxation on cigarettes—combined with restrictions on smoking in public places. This has led to calls for taxing unhealthy foods, yet governments have been remarkably resistant to that suggestion. Cancer prevention interventions, if fully implemented, could potentially prevent several hundred thousand cancer deaths per year, but if this is to be achieved much of the emphasis should be on children, as most prevention interventions are most useful when deployed early in life. Effective interventions must be applied at the individual, clinical, community, and policy levels—a public health challenge at national and local levels. Controlling the causes of cancer requires a coordinated effort for the identification of exposed populations, particularly in low-income countries, and for effective primary prevention policies.

Several strategies have been proposed for reducing the incidence of cancer. These include scaling up preventive maneuvers in primary care settings, introducing high-reach, low-cost programs (using print and electronic media), and creating environments that promote healthy behaviour patterns. Given the importance of tobacco use in inducing cancer and other chronic diseases, in the future, in addition to more effective measures that will influence individual behaviour, tobacco control may need to be expanded to include measures directed at changing the ways tobacco suppliers do business, in effect by ensuring that governments take control of supply and progressively reduce that supply. We know that controlling cancer-causing occupational exposures leads to a reduction in cancer risk, but information is needed to identify and characterise successful exposure-reduction approaches to reduce the cancer burden on all working populations in a timely manner. As well, action to prevent the exportation of cancer-causing agents (such as asbestos) and occupations to developing countries would reduce occupationally induced cancer in those countries.

It is now believed that infections are responsible for 15% of cancers the world over, and it is possible that some behavioural changes in infected individuals, such as smoking cessation, alcohol abstinence (in patients with chronic hepatitis B and C), and reduction of salt intake (in *H. pylori* carriers) can reduce the corresponding cancer risks. We also believe that comprehensive strategies of HPV vaccination and HPV-based screening tests could eliminate cervical cancer in defined populations, thus profiting on the knowledge that infection with cancer-causing types of HPV is a necessary cause of cancer of the cervix.

Physical activity is a modifiable lifestyle risk factor associated with a decreased risk of several cancers, especially of the breast and colon, although sedentary behaviour is emerging as a risk factor for cancer that should be considered independently from physical

activity. Evidence is growing that the contribution of diet in the causation of cancer has previously been underestimated. An emphasis
on the components of a healthy diet, especially fruit and vegetable
consumption, less dietary fat, and less red and processed meat is
needed, as is attention to healthy diets in cancer survivors.

It is now recognised that women should be informed that early
age at the birth of one's first child protects against breast cancer, and
that risk of both breast and ovarian cancers declines with increasing
duration of breastfeeding.

It is also now recognized that although early detection of all
cancers is important for improved survival, the possible role of
screening for many cancers has been over-emphasised. Screening for
cancer of the uterine cervix is an effective way to reduce deaths from
the disease, but there are many challenges for cervical cancer control
programs. These include the need to reform health care systems
in many countries and ensure the availability of human resources
because of a shortage of health workers trained to vaccinate, screen,
and treat identified lesions. However it has been demonstrated in
Finland that screening for cervical cancer can be relatively inex-
pensive and highly effective if coverage of the total target population is achieved. An important future influence on screening for
cervix cancer will be vaccination against HPV infection, although
screening for cervix cancer will continue to have an important role.
Although colon screening can be expensive, depending on the test
used, any type of screening appears to be cost-effective. However,
we may have reached the point of negligible benefit in screening for invasive breast cancer, largely because of improvements in
cancer therapy. Similarly, there seems to be no justification for the
introduction of population-based organized screening for prostate
cancer at any age, while, in view of the potential harms associated
with screening, physicians should generally recommend against
PSA testing for asymptomatic men. In many respects these contrasting conclusions on screening reflect the fact that when screening for a precursor, as for cervix and colon cancer, removal of the

precursor results in reduction in both incidence and mortality from the cancer, whereas when screening for the cancer when a precursor is not known, the absolute benefit in terms of mortality reduction declines drastically as treatment improves.

One of the major challenges for cancer control the world over is the continuing burden of lung cancer, increasingly in developing countries, largely because of lack of restrictions in such countries of the activities of the tobacco industry. It is possible that the combination of low-dose computerized tomography and, in the future, biomarkers, will help improve the accuracy and clinical utility of lung screening programs, although all screening programs should incorporate access to tobacco cessation resources. Asia has the largest cancer burden of any region in the world but knowledge of cancer prevention and early detection could make major inroads into reducing the cancer burden. In nearly every country primary care practitioners should have a major role in educating patients and supporting lifestyle changes to reduce exposure to cancer risk factors. Family practice has a key role in cancer prevention and in targeting of specific populations for screening.

There is, therefore, a great deal that can be done to raise the profile of cancer prevention and to ensure that approaches to early detection and screening do not consume resources that could be more effectively used for cancer prevention. Too frequently National Cancer Control Programs are initiated without the benefit of prior strategic planning to ensure that available resources are appropriately used. Governments need to take a longer-term view as to what is possible and what can be accomplished. All components of government are potentially involved, not just ministries of health but also those concerned with agriculture, finance, and social security.

But, most critically, the prevention of cancer is dependent upon individuals in every community who understand about cancer and are prepared to be an exemplar of good practices and role models for their families and friends. This book has been primarily dedicated to facilitating this critical role.

23535235235235525352355

Resources

It is impossible to list all my sources as this book is based upon almost a lifetime of research into the causes of cancer and its control. However, I have made liberal use of the international databases established by the International Agency for Research on Cancer (www.iarc.fr), on cancer incidence from cancer registries, on cancer mortality from the World Health Organization mortality data base, and Globocan, which provides estimates of the numbers of cancer cases and deaths worldwide, the latest at the time of writing being for 2012. I have consulted the book *Cancer Epidemiology and Prevention*, Second Edition, edited by David Schottenfeld and Joseph F. Fraumeni, Jr. (New York Oxford University Press, 1996), and have updated from my extensive reading of the literature much of what is stated on the causation of cancer. I have also drawn on a book I edited, *Epidemiologic Studies in Cancer Prevention and Screening: Statistics for Biology and Health*; Volume 79. Springer Verlag, New York, 2013. ISBN: 978-1-4614-5585-1 (print) 978-1-4614-5586-8 (digital).

Another useful authoritative resource that can be found online is the US National Library of Medicine *PubMed Health* (www.ncbi.nlm.nih.gov). This has information that extends to the symptomatology of the cancer, information I have not included in this book as my purpose was to concentrate on our understanding of the causes of the cancers considered.